Astrology
for
Layman

Dr. T.M. Rao
B.Sc. (Hons.), M.Sc. (Research), D.Sc. (Colombo)
Astrologer

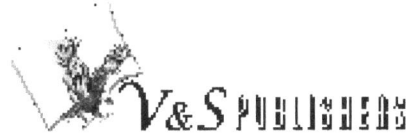

Published by:

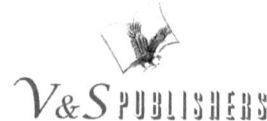

F-2/16, Ansari Road, Daryaganj, New Delhi-110002
☎ 011-23240026, 011-23240027 • *Fax:* 011-23240028
Email: info@vspublishers.com • *Website:* www.vspublishers.com

Regional Office : Hyderabad
5-1-707/1, Brij Bhawan (Beside Central Bank of India Lane)
Bank Street, Koti, Hyderabad - 500 095
☎ 040-24737290
E-mail: vspublishershyd@gmail.com

Branch Office : Mumbai
Godown # 34 at The Model Co-Operative Housing, Society Ltd.,
"Sahakar Niwas", Ground Floor, Next to Sobo Central, Mumbai - 400 034
☎ 022-23510736
E-mail vspublishersmum@gmail.com

Follow us on:

All books available at **www.vspublishers.com**

© **Copyright:** V&S PUBLISHERS
ISBN 978-93-813843-7-4
Edition 2014

The Copyright of this book, as well as all matter contained herein (including illustrations) rests with the Publisher. No person shall copy the name of the book, its title design, matter and illustrations in any form and in any language, totally or partially or in any form. Anybody doing so shall face legal action and will be responsible for damages.

Printed at : Param Offseters Okhla New Delhi-110020

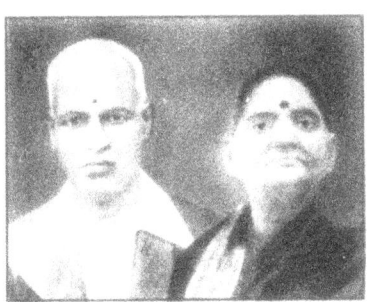

Dedication

This work is dedicated respectfully to the memory of my late parents Shri Turaga Ramayya (Father) and Smt. Turaga Sriranganaiki Devi (Mother)

Contents

Preface	7
1. General Principles	9
2. Planets' Characteristics	19
3. Casting of Lagna and Other Details	25
4. Planetary Strength	29
5. Span of Life	34
6. Rasi Effects	37
7. On Bhavas	42
8. Planets and Signs	58
9. The Position of Bhavadhipathis in Houses	65
10. Some Important Points	77
11. Dasa Periods	81
12. Yogas	96
13. Issue	104
14. Matrimony	107
15. Female Horoscope	117
16. Health and Planets	122
17. Profession	130
18. Gochara (Transit)	135
19. Hora	145
20. Death	147
21. Muhurta or Election	157
22. Prayers	159
23. Birth Star Significance	164
24. Hindu Time Measure	166
Conclusion	174
References	176

Preface

The title of the book itself speaks that it is intended for the Laymen who are not conversant with much of Mathematical study.

Astrology is a portion of Veda. The ancient sages brought out wonderful thoughts regarding planets and their significance. Many do not know past Karma. Then what is the analysis for one person who is rich and powerful and the other who is poor and downtrodden. Man is born again and again to reap his Karma only till he attains Atma Gyana. The previous Karma is determined by the part played at the time of birth.

Several astrologers give several kinds of opinions for a horoscope. Each feels he is right in his own way. This kind of too many opinions are not peculiar to this branch alone. Swamy Sivananda used to say, when there is one Doctor there is one prescription, when two there is consultation and when three it is cremation. In medical field, Vedanta, in scientific theories, in literature there are many schools of thought.

Basic factors do not change. This book is for the Layman who is to be guided to understand the fundamentals of astrology. In order to meet this need and to enable the readers to understand the scope and extend their talents to research and investigation the benefits have been described.

All the necessary and useful information has been treated with great care and study. This book is intended for the Layman as all the details needed for scientifically deciphering the future have been fully described with emphasis on elementary portions so essential for the Layman.

One who reads this book carefully and dispassionately will understand the principles incorporated, will not only be able to make fairly correct predictions but will be encouraged to take to the study of more advanced works and thus help the cause of this science.

As a science astrology has discovered correct methods and knowledge about the influence of planets on the human mind and on the day to day activities of the human beings.

In the pages that follow, I have in my own humble way attempted to bring to the fore not only the rationality of astrology but also the nature and structure of the correct knowledge that our forefathers possessed regarding the predictable influences of planets on human beings, and to give a spiritual bias to astrology. The reader is led step by step in this work, from the rudiments to the final stage of reading the brighter and darker side of the subject life, his chances of success and failure.

The aim of astrology is to dispel the fear of the unknown and to give scope for the fair play of the human system. This treatise is not complete by any means. The subject is vast, yet I have gathered information and culled the relevant portions from the acknowledged sources. I am sure this information will be of great use to the common-man, with the help of this book, he would be able to exercise his own judgement.

I take this opportunity to express my heartfelt thanks to M/s. Pustak Mahal for their suggestion on writing this book.

If the reader should be enabled, by study of this book to acquire a working knowledge of astrology, my labours will have been amply rewarded.

T.M. Rao

1. General Principles

Nobody need be ashamed of entertaining a desire to learn the ancient subject of astrology. The thirst for knowledge is a legitimate ambition of human beings. Astrology is not a forbidden fruit. To Hindus especially, it is one of their Sacred Sciences or Sastras. For it is reckoned as one of the limbs of the Vedas. The predictive part of astrology is as scientific as the mathematical one, as the former is directly based upon the latter. Moreover, ancient sages had discovered the truth of predictive astrology through their meditation or penance and intuitional perception. All the authors of Dharma Sastras and host of other poets and seers like Vyasa, Valmiki, Kalidasa have cherished and developed this science of astrology which is one of the cornerstones of Indian Culture. So, if you have any regard for culture as such, you must necessarily pay your homage to this science. In ancient India astrologers were held in high esteem, as they combined both a scientific bent of mind and a spiritual outlook on life as well as a pure life of high moral standard. They practised this lore not for amassing wealth, but for giving guidance to the needy and distressed. Their aim was to remove the cause of suffering among the people and to turn their minds towards Dharma and God. Hence, a reverential attitude is expected of the students of astrology.

According to the Indian system there are nine planets i.e. the seven planets whose names are attached to the week days and Rahu and Ketu. Their English names are Sun, Moon, Mars, Mercury, Jupiter, Venus, Saturn, Dragon's Head or Ascending Node, and Dragon's Tail or Descending Node. The Zodiac which is a circle has twelve Rasis or Signs which the planets traverse during their journey. These Rasis are called (1) Mesha - *Aries*, (2) Vrishabha - *Taurus*, (3) Mithuna - *Gemini*, (4) Karkataka or Kataka - *Cancer*, (5) Simha - *Leo*,

(6) Kanya - *Virgo*, (7) Tula - *Libra*, (8) Vrischika - *Scorpio*, (9) Dhanus - *Sagittarius*, (10) Makara - *Capricorn* (11) Kumbha - *Aquarius* and (12) Meena - *Pisces*

Meena 12	Mesha 1	Vrishabha 2	Mithuna 3
Kumbha 11			Karkataka 4
Makara 10			Simha 5
Dhanus 9	Vrischika 8	Tula 7	Kanya 6

Fig. I

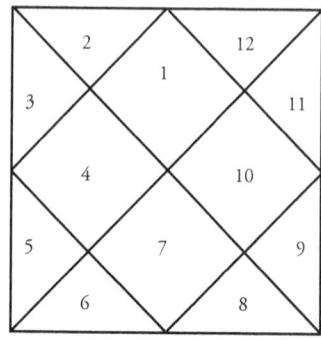

Fig. II

Figure II shows the chart as drawn in North India. The difference between the two is that in the South Indian chart the position of several rasis never change, whereas in the other the lagna or Ascendent is put at the top and counting is done in the opposite direction. In the South Indian chart too the people of coastal Andhra, Orissa and West Bengal also show in the opposite direction and it is called **apasavya**. Predominantly people of South India, Madras, Kerala and Karnatak follow the clockwise one i.e. **savya** (Fig. I). But in practice, it is very convenient to follow the savya charts. So some astrologers convert the apasavya charts to savya charts and study them to avoid confusion. The apasavya chart is given below:

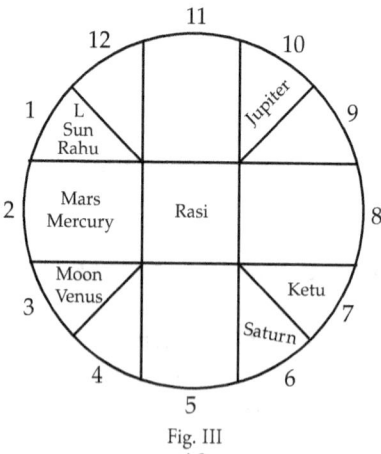

Fig. III

In fig. III, the reckoning is from Mesha itself and it remains stationary and the counting is done anticlockwise and house no. 1 is always the lagna or the ascendant. In fig. III the lagna is Mithuna and the other signs follow. Likewise it has to be adhered for other lagnas.

Now the belt of zodiac contains 27 constellations or Nakshtras distributed among the 12 Rasis beginning from Mesha. If you divide 27 by 12, you get 2 . So each Rasi contains two stars and a quarter. In other words, each Sign contains nine padas or quarters of stars. Mesha has Aswini, Bharani and the first pada of Krittika, Vrishabha the remaining three quarters of Krittika, Rohini and the first two padas of Mrigasira; Mithuna, the latter half of Mrigasira, Aridra, and the first three quarters of Punarvasu; Karkataka, the last pada of Punarvasu, Pushyami, and the whole of Aslesha Simha, Makha, Purva Phalguni (Pubba) and the first pada of Uttara Phalguni (Uttara); Kanya, the remaining three padas of Uttara Phalguni, Hastha, and the first half of Chitta; Tula, the latter half of Chitta Swathi, and the first three quarters of Visakha, Vrischika, the last quarter of Visakha, Anuradha and the whole of Jeysta; Dhanus, Moola, Poorvashada and the first of Uttarashada; Makara, the remaining three quarters of Uttarashada, Sravana, and the first half of Dhanista Kumbha, the latter half of Dhanista, Satabhisham, and the first three padas of Purvabhadra; and Meena, the last quarter of Purvabhadra, Uttarabhadra and Revathi. The diagram given on the next page clearly shows the same.

The Divine Sun is the King and the Ruler of the Planetary kingdom. The moon is his Consort. So the whole zodiac of 12 signs belong to the Divine Royal Couple. The Sun is ruling over the six signs beginning with Simha and ending with Makara. His queen, the Moon, was ruling over six signs from Karkataka, counting being done in anticlockwise manner. The idea is that the Sun and the Moon were living in their respective palaces viz. Simha and Karkataka and ruling over their respective domains. The couple was noted for their generosity. So each one of the remaining planets, Rahu and Ketu excepted, went to these

Meena *(Pisces)* Revathi - 4 U. Bhadra - 4 P. Bhadra - 4	Mesha *(Aries)* Aswini - 4 Bharani - 4 Krittika - 1	Vrishabha *(Taurus)* Krittika - 3 Rohini - 4 Mrigasira - 2	Mithuna *(Gemini)* Mrigasira-2 Aridra - 4 Punarvasu - 3
Kumbha *(Aquarius)* P. Bhadra-3 Satabhisam - 4 Dhanista - 3,4	Each pada - 3 20' Each Rasi - 2 stars Each Star - 4 padas Each Sign - 30		Kataka *(Cancer)* Punarvasu - 1 Pushyami - 4 Aslesha - 4
Makara *(Capricorn)* Dhanista-1,2 Sravanam-4 U. Ashada-2,3,4			Simha *(Leo),* Makha-4, P. Phalguni-4 U. Phalguni-1
Dhanus *(Sagittarius)* U. Ashada-1, P. Ashada-4, Moola-4	Vrischika *(Scorpio)* Visakha-4 Anuradha-4 Jyesta-4	Tula *(Libra)* Chitta-3,4 Swathi-4 Visakha-1,2,3	Kanya *(Virgo)* U. Phalguni-3 Hastha-4 Chitta-2

luminaries to ask for a house to occupy. For, it is natural for a houseless person to wish to have a house to live in. At first Mercury who is closest to Sun went to him and begged him for a house. Out of pure compassion he gave him a house i.e. Rasi next to him i.e. Kanya. Mercury was not satisfied with one. So, he quietly went to the Moon and repeated the request without telling her that he had already got a house from the King. The Moon too gave a house to Mercury next to her i.e. Mithuna. That is how Budha came to have two houses, Kanya and Mithuna. This news reached Sukra, Kuja, Guru and Sani also. So they too one after the other played the same trick and each one got two houses, leaving only one house to each of the luminaries i.e. Sun and Moon. Thus Venus became the lord of Tula and Vrishabha (positive and negative) Mars, Vrischika and Mesha (negative and positive), Guru, Dhanus and Meena (positive and negative) and lastly Saturn, Makara and

Kumbha (negative and positive). The signs are divided into odd and even. The odd signs are Aries, Gemini, Leo, Libra, Sagittarius and Aquarius and are called Krura or fierce, while the even Rasis viz. Tauras, Cancer, Virgo, Scorpio, Capricorn and Pisces are called Saumya or gentle. The odd and even signs are also called as Male and Female ones respectively. Make the 12 rasis into 4 groups of three rasis each. So the first group would consist of Mesha, Vrishabha and Mithuna. They are called in order Chara, or moveable, Sthira or fixed and Dwisambhava or common signs. Repeat this order with regard to other groups as well. You know that a circle has 360 degrees at its centre. So if a circle is divided into 12 parts or sectors each would get 30 degrees. Thus you see that a Rasi or Sign consists of 30 degrees.

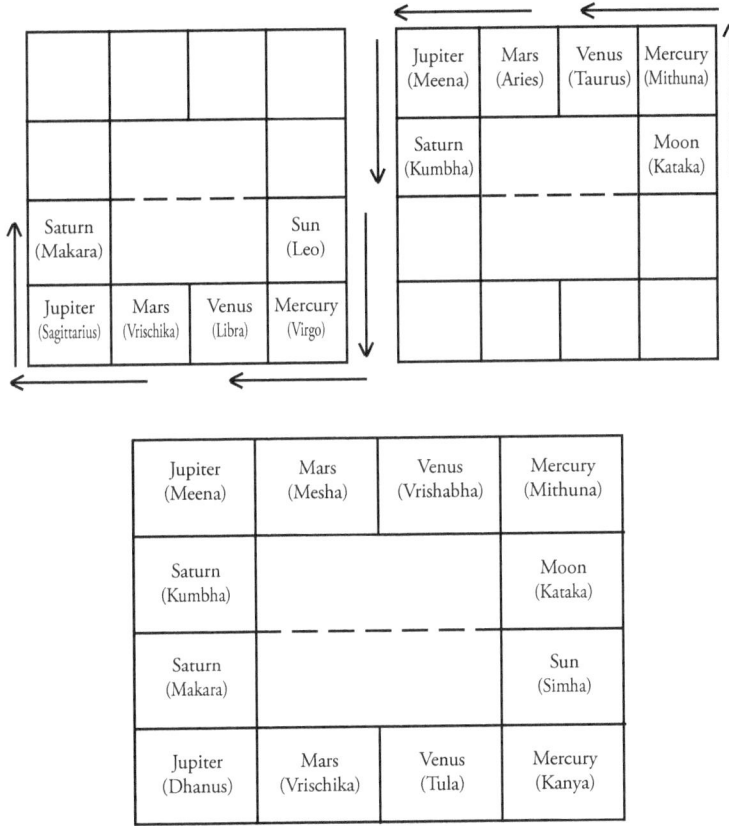

	even	odd	even	odd	
FM	Meena Jupiter Dwisambhava	Chara Mesha Mars	Sthira Vrishabha Venus	Dwisambhava Mithuna Mercury	M
odd M	Kumbha Saturn Sthira	M		Chara Kataka Moon	even FM
even FM	Makara Saturn Chara		FM	Sthira Simha Sun	odd M
	Dhanus Jupiter Dwisambhava	Vrischika Mars Sthira	Tula Venus Chara	Kanya Mercury Dwisambhava	Even
	M odd	even FM	odd M	FM	

M = MALE
FM = FEMALE

The odd signs are—Aries, Gemini, Leo, Libra, Sagittarius and Aquarius. The even rasis are—Taurus, Cancer, Virgo, Scorpio, Capricorn and Pisces.

Similarly the Male rasis are—Mesha, Mithuna, Simha, Tula, Dhanus and Kumbha. The Female rasis are— Vrishabha Kataka, Kanya, Vrischika, Makara, and Meena.

The Chara rasis are—Mesha, Kataka, Tula, Makara.

The Sthira rasis are—Vrishabha, Simha, Vrischika, Kumbha.

The Dwisambhava rasis are—Mithuna, Kanya, Dhanur and Meena.

Hora: Such a rasi is first divided into two equal parts or halves called Horas. So each Hora measures 15 degrees. Who are the owners of these Horas in the several signs? They are divided into only two planets viz. the Sun and the Moon. There is some difference. In all odd signs viz. Mesha, Simha, Tula, Dhanus and Kumbha, the first Hora is ruled by the Sun and the second by the Moon, while in the even signs this order is reversed i.e. the first belongs to Moon and the next to the Sun. Thus you see that in all there are 24 Horas in the Zodiac and out of them 12 are held by the Sun and the remaining 12 by the Moon.

Drekkana: A Rasi is further divided into three equal parts of 10 degrees each. Each part is named as Drekkana or Decante. In each sign the first Decante is owned by the lord of the same Sign, the second by the lord of the 5th Rasi from that and the third by the lord of the 9th sign from the original one. For example in Mesha, the first Drekkana is called the Mesha itself, and its lord should be Mars, the second Simha is ruled by the sun and the third by the Dhanus owned by Jupiter. In this manner you can easily find out the decantes of all the Rasis.

Navamsa: A sign is further divided into nine equal parts called Navamsa. What is the measure of a Navamsa? It is 30 degree divided by 9. This is equal to $^{10}/_3$ degrees or 3 degrees and 20 minutes. Now we must see how these navamsas are counted in the several Rasis. In respect of this we have to make four groups of three rasis each as follows: (1) Mesha, Simha and Dhanus, (2) Vrishabha, Kanya and Makara, (3) Mithuna, Tula and Kumbha, and (4) Karkataka Vrischika and Meena. In the first group the Navamsas begin with Mesha and end with Dhanus. In other words the first Navamsa of Mesha, Simha and Dhanus will be mesha itself, and the last Dhanus. In the second group the Navamsa begins with Makara and end with Kanya. In other words the first Navamsa or Vrishabha, Kanya and Makara is Makara and the last Kanya. So the first Navamsa of the Makara is the same and the last of Kanya is Kanya itself. But the Vrishabha-Navamsa of Vrishabha rasi is neither the first nor the last. It is the 5th Navamsa. In this manner if you work out you will see that a particular Navamsa bears the same name as the Rasi itself. In the third group Navamsa begins with Tula and ends with Mithuna. So the first Navamsa of Tula is Tula itself, and the last of Mithuna is Mithuna itself. Lastly the Navamsa of the fourth group of Rasis begin with Karkataka itself and the last of Meena is Meena itself. In this manner you can see that in every Rasi there is a Navamsa which bears the same name. In other words both the Rasi and Navamsa have the same lord. It is now clear that in all the Chara Rasis the Navamsa bears the same names are the first ones, in all the Sthira Rasis they are the 5th, and in all Dwisambhava or Common signs they are the last or the 9th.

A sign consists of 2 stars of 9 quarter stars. So you can easily equate a Navamsa with a quarter star.

Dwadasamsa: A Rasi is further divided into 12 equal parts termed Dwadasamsa, each subdivision getting an angle of 2/1/4 degrees. Regarding the names of these 12 parts there is absolutely no difficulty, as the Dwadasamsa in each Rasi begins with the same Rasi and end with the one that is 12th from it. That is to say, in Mesha the 12 parts are counted from Mesha onwards ending in Meena, in Vrishabha the first part is Vrishabha itself and the last Mesha and so on.

Trisamsa: This is nothing but a one degree position of a Rasi. Hence there should be 30 such parts or degree portions belonging to 30 planets, which is an impossibility. Their lords are only the five planets viz: Mars, Mercury, Jupiter, Venus and Saturn. The Sun and the Moon have no play in this. With regard to the distribution of these degrees there is a difference in respect of odd and even rasis. In the odd signs i.e. 1,3,5,7, 9 and 11 the distribution is as follows: The first 5 degrees belong to Mars, the next 5 degrees to Saturn, next 8 to Jupiter, the next 7 to Mercury and the last 5 to Venus. In an even sign this order is reversed: The first 5 degrees go to Venus, the next 7 to Mercury, the next 8 to Jupiter, the next 5 to Saturn and the last 5 to Mars.

So far I have explained to you about six vargas viz: Rasi, Hora, Drekkana, Navamsa, Dwdasamsa and Trisamsa. These six are called **Shadvargas**. Please bear this in mind as it is one of the fundamental principles of this science.

Characteristics of the Rasis: The forms of the twelve signs beginning with Mesha are in order (1) a Ram, (2) a Bull, (3) a Human Couple of which the man holds a staff and the woman a lute-*Vina* (4) a Crab, (5) a Lion, (6) a Maiden seated in a boat holding fire and green plant, (7) a Man holding scales, (8) a Scorpio, (9) a Man holding a bow and having the body of a horse beneath the hips,

(10) a Crocodile with the face of a deer, (11) a Man holding a pot, and (12) a pair of Fish. Signs Kataka, Vrischika, Makar and Meena are termed watery ones as well as aquatic (moving in water); Vrishabha, Kanya, Tula and Kumbha are called jalasrayas or dependant upon water and delighting in places abounding in water, and the remaining rasis viz. Mesha, Mithuna, Simha and Dhanus, are land signs. Kataka or Karkataka, Vrischika and Meena are also termed Kitas or Reptiles. This appellation is mostly applied to Vrischika.

Do not be under the impression that all the signs rise in the same manner. Some rise with their heads first and some other with their hind parts foremost. Mesha, Vrishabha, Karkataka, Dhanus and Makara rise with their hind parts first, while Simha, Kanya, Tula, Vrischika and Kumbha rise with their heads foremost. Mithuna and Meena rise both ways, because their two constituents face each other. The Sanskrit names for these three types of Rasis are respectively (1) Pristodaya, (2) Srishodaya and (3) Ubhayodaya.

Those signs coming under the category of Sivodayas, six in all, ruled by the Sun are called Diurnal Signs, while the Pristodayas and Mithuna come under the Moon and so are called Nocturnal ones. Sign Meena is a twilight—Sandhya Sign.

The colours of the twelve signs are in order (1) Red (2) White, (3) Green, (4) Pink, (5) Brown, (6) Grey, (7) Variegated, (8) Black, (9) Golden, (10) Yellow, (11) Variegated, and (12) Deep Brown.

Aquarious, Pisces, Aries, and Taurus are short, Gemini Cancer, Sagittarius and Capricorn are of medium length, and Leo, Virgo, Libra and Scorpio, long.

Kalapurusha's Limbs:

The whole zodiac consists of the twelve signs representing the Body of the Supreme being termed Kala or Time. The twelve signs, therefore, stand for head, face, neck, arms, heart, stomach, abdomen, private parts, thighs, knees, shanks and feet respectively of Kalapurusha.

When a horoscope is made, you will find therein a

certain Rasi being put as Lagna or Ascendant. What does it mean? You know zodiac is like a wheel. It appears to revolve as time passes on. So the Rasis rise, as does the Sun, above the horizon one after the other. Thus at the time of birth one of the signs will be rising above the horizon. That is called as Lagna. We have to begin with the Lagna as the starting point. In other words the Lagna will represent the head of the Native and the next house his face and so on. This will be explained in due course as to how to calculate Lagna etc.

2. Planets' Characteristics

We have already learnt about the Rasis and their lords. The planets wield different kinds of authority over the Rasis they are connected with. Mesha is called the Exaltation - *Ucha* house of the Sun, although that house belongs to Mars. It means the Sun is very strong in that house. Similarly the Ucha Rasis of the remaining six planets are respectively, Vrishabha, Makara, Kanya, Karkataka, Meena and Tula. Though these are the Exaltation houses, yet there is a particular degree in them which is termed the Highest Exaltation point. So for the 7 planets beginning with the Sun the degree of highest exaltation are in order–10th, 3rd, 28th, 15th, 5th, 27th and 20th in their respective exaltation Rasis. So, one can call the Sun really exalted if he is in the 10th degree of Mesha. On the other hand if he is in the 20th degree of the same sign, you could only say that he is in his exaltation sign but not in his highest exaltation, as he has fallen from that point. There must be a Rasi where a planet is debilitated i.e. *Neecha*, also. Yes, the house 7th from the exaltation sign is called Debilitation Sign of a planet. So what is the Neecha Rasi for Sun? It must be Tula as it is the 7th from Mesha. In the same manner one can easily find out the Neecha houses for the other planets. They are in order, Vrischika, Karkataka, Meena, Makara, Kanya and Mesha. In this also there is the lowest debilitation which is the same for exaltation. Thus, the Sun is in his lowest debilitation if he is in the 10th degree of Tula. You can now find out which pada of the Nakshatra has this highest exaltation or lowest debilitation. The former will be in the third quarter of Aswini and the latter in the first pada of Swathi. Another aspect of this subject is the relationship between the Sun and Saturn, Mars and Jupiter and Mercury and Venus. For the exaltation of one is the debilitation of the other and vice versa.

Mulatrikona: In addition to exaltation and debilitation signs, there is another house called Mulatrikona house. The Sun's own house is Simha. This is his Mulatrikona also. One may find it difficult to distinguish between the two kinds of houses. So there is a way out for this dilemma, the initial 20 degrees portion of Simha is called his Mulatrikona, and the last 10 degrees his own house or Swakshetra. So if Sun is anywhere between the beginning of the Simha and 20 degrees portion of Simha, one should say that he is in his Mulatrikona. Beyond that point one has to say that he is in his Swakshetra or own House. In Vrishabha the first 3 degrees constitute the Moon's exaltation portion and the remaining 27 degrees is her Mulatrikona. In Mesha the initial 12 degrees is the Mulatrikona of Mars and the remaining 18 degrees his Swakshetra. Vrischika is therefore his Swakshetra only, negative house. For Budha the first half i.e. 15 degrees of Kanya is his Exaltation. Beyond that portion upto 20 degrees is his Mulatrikona, and the last 10 degrees are his Swakshetra. Thus in the one sign you see three types of relationship. Mithuna is his positive swakshetra. In Dhanus the first 5 degrees constitute the Mulatriokna of Guru and the rest his own house. In Tula the initial 20 degrees are the Mulatrikona of venus and the rest own house. Lastly in Kumbha the first 20 degrees constitute Saturn's Mulatrikona and the rest own house. Now you can ask about Rahu and Ketu. Rahu is considered strong in Karkataka, Vrishabha, Mesha, Kumbha and Vrischika while ketu is strong in Meena, Kanya, Vrishabha and the latter half of Dhanus. There is much difference of opinion about this. Rahu's Swakshetra is supposed to be Kanya, Mulatrikonas are Mithuna and Karkataka and exaltation is Vrishabha. Ketu's Swakshetra is Meena, Mulatrikona is Dhanus and exaltation Vrischika. According to another version Rahu is exalted in Mithuna, has Simha as his Mulatrikona and Kanya as Swakshetra. Ketu is Exalted in Dhanus, has Kumbha as Mulatrikona and Meena as Swakshetra.

Sex of planets: The Sun, Mars and Jupiter are males,

the Moon, Venus and Rahu females, and Mercury, Saturn and Ketu eunuchs.

Castes of planets: Jupiter and Venus are Brahmins, the Sun and Mars are Kshatriyas, the Moon Vaisya, Mercury of mixed caste, Saturn Sudra and Rahu an outcaste. According to another view Mercury is a Sudra and Saturn an outcaste. There is yet another view according to which Mercury is a Vaisya.

Their nature: Mercury, Jupiter and Venus are naturally benevolent. Similarly the waxing Moon is a benefic. The waning Moon and Mercury with a malefic are malefics. The Sun, Mars, Saturn, Rahu and Ketu are naturally malevolent.

Their qualities: The Sun, Moon and Jupiter are of *Satvika* (pure or good) nature, Mercury and Venus of *Rajasa* (active, passionate) nature, and the rest viz. Mars, Saturn, Rahu and Ketu of Tamasa (dark, ignorant) nature.

Humours: The Sun and Mars have pitta or bile as the chief humour of their body; the Moon and Venus Vata or wind and Kapha or phlegm; Saturn Vata or wind, Mercury a mixture of all the three humours; and Jupiter Kapha or phlegm.

Seasons: There are six seasons or Ritus viz. Vasanta, (Spring), Grisma (Summer), Varsha (Rainy), Sarad (Autumn), Hemanta (Dewy) and Sisira (Winter). These belong to (1) Venus, (2) the Sun, and Mars, (3) Moon, (4) Mercury, (5) Jupiter and (6) Saturn respectively. Note that there are two lords for Summer.

Their gems: Sun's precious stone is Manikya or ruby, the Moon's Pearl, Mar's Coral, Mercury's Marakata or emerald, Jupiter's Pushyaraga or topaz, Venus' Diamond, Saturn's Neelam, Rahu's Gomedhika or agate, and Ketu's Vaidhurya or lapis lazuli.

Their grains: The grains owned by the 9 planets are in order (1) Wheat (2) Rice (3) Adhaka or Tuvar (4) Green gram (5) Bengal gram (6) Cow gram (7) Sesamum (8) Black gram and (9) Horse gram.

Presiding deities: The nine deities are in order (1) Rudra or Siva (2) the Divine Mother, Parvati (3) Kartikeya (4) Vishnu (5) Brahman (or Siva) (6) Lakshmi (7) Kala or Yamuna (or Rudra) (8) Adisesha King of serpents (or Kartikeya) and (9) Brahman (or Vighneshwara).

Physical constituents: In Ayurveda seven Dhatus (matter) are spoken of as constituting the Body. They are (1) Bones (2) Blood (3) Marrow (4) Skin (5) Fat (6) Semen and (7) Muscles. These are respectively presided over by the seven planets beginning with the Sun.

Elements: There are five elements constituting the entire Universe. They are (1) Prithvi or Earth (2) Apah or water (3) Teja or Fire (4) Vayu or Wind and (5) Akasha or Ether. Do not confuse these things with the visible earth etc. These are the subtle things of which you see the grosser forms in the world. The Sun and Mars own fire, the Moon and Venus water, Mercury earth, Jupiter ether and Saturn wind.

Planetary cabinet: The Sun and Moon are the Royal Couple, Mars the Commander, Mercury the Crown Prince, Jupiter and Venus are Ministers and Saturn the Servant. These seven planets also represent in order Soul, Mind, Courage, Speech, Wisdom, Happiness, Sexual passion and grief. They also represent the senses and their functions thus–Mercury governs smell (nose), the Moon and Venus the taste (tongue), the Sun and Mars form (eye) Jupiter sound (ear) and Saturn, Rahu and Ketu touch (skin).

Planetary aspects: The planets have four kinds of aspects. The mode of looking at the 3rd and 10th houses from the one occupied by a planet is termed a quarter aspect, looking at the 5th and 9th is half-aspect at the 4th and 8th houses is aspect and at the 7th house is full aspect. There is a speciality in the case of Jupiter, Mars and Saturn. In the case of Saturn even the quarter aspect is considered to be full. So, he aspects fully at the 3rd, 7th and 10th house from the house occupied by him. In case of Jupiter even half aspect is considered to be full. So he aspects fully the 5th, 7th and 9th houses from the house occupied by him. In the case of Mars even a aspect is full. So he aspects fully the 4th,

7th and 8th houses from the house occupied by him. You know that Mars and Saturn are among Malefics. Hence their aspects cannot but be malevolent in nature.

Their friends: As we have best friends, ordinary friends, neutrals, enemies and inveterate foes, so do planets in their life. The following table gives the friends, neutrals and enemies of the several planets.

Planets	Friends	Enemies	Neutrals
Sun	Moon, Mars & Jupiter	Venus and Saturn	Mercury
Moon	Sun and Mercury	Nil	The rest.
Mars	Sun, Moon and Jupiter	Mercury	Venus and Saturn.
Mercury	Sun and Venus	Moon	Mars, Jupt. & Saturn
Jupiter	Sun, Moon and Mars	Mercury & Venus	Saturn
Venus	Mercury & Saturn	Sun & Moon	Mars & Jupt
Saturn	Mercury & Venus	Sun, Moon & Mars	Jupiter
Rahu & Ketu	Mercury, Saturn & Venus	Sun, Moon & Jupt	Mars.

According to others Rahu is the enemy of the Sun, Moon and Mars, neutral to Jupiter, while ketu is neutral to Mercury. In case of friendship and enemity Rahu and Ketu are in opposite camp. However, it is always believed that Rahu and Ketu are shadow planets and are generally malevolent in nature.

The Sun and other planets are called as Karakas or Significators of certain relatives of the native: father, mother, younger brother, maternal uncle, children, wife or husband and servant are signified in order by the seven planets. There are many other things for which these planets are Karakas too. For the present this will suffice. Rahu and Ketu indicate maternal and paternal grandfathers respectively.

Please remember that every planet is strong in its own house etc. mentioned above.

Venus 27°	Sun 10°	Moon 3°	
	Exaltation 5° houses of planets		Jupiter
Mars 28°			
		Saturn 20°	Mercury 15°

Mercury 15°	Saturn 20°		
	Debilitation houses of planets		Mars 28°
Jupiter 5°			
	Moon 3°	Sun 10°	Venus 27°

	Mars	Moon	
Saturn	Moola Trikona Houses		
			Sun
Jupiter		Venus	Mercury

Aspects (Jupiter)

Aspects (Mars)

Aspects (Saturn)

3. Casting of Lagna and Other Details

When watches were not available, people used to find out time of birth from the shadows at daytime, and from the stars in the heavens at night. Now that we have watches of all varieties the difficulty of looking into the above methods is obviated. So what one has to do to start with is to ascertain the correct time of birth (the first cry of the baby) as well as the place and date of birth. Then have before you Lahiri's Tables of Ascendants' and the Ephemeris for the year. The ascendant (lagna) and other houses vary according to the altitude of the place. To calculate the lagna you have to convert the time in I.S.T. to the Local Mean Time which one can read from the pages of the Lahiri's Ephemeris. For example you find against Delhi: Latitude 28.39; Longitude 77.13; Local time correction to Indian Standard Time (I.S.T.) minus 21 m (minute) 8 s (second) and lastly correction to Indian Siderial Time +3s. Hence you will deduct 21 m and 8 S from the I.S.T. in order to get the Local Mean Time i.e. L.M.T. at Delhi. You will also find for each day of the year the Siderial time at Noon, correction to which is given above as plus 3 seconds. Then you will find the Siderial Time for the moment of the birth. This is worked out thus–Find the difference between the L.M.T. and the noon i.e. 12 hours. It is minus if the L.M.T. is before noon and plus if it is after the noon. The Siderial equivalent of this difference is obtained by adding to it 10 seconds per hour. If the birth is before noon, deduct the siderial equivalent from the Siderial time at noon, if it is afternoon, add it to the S.T. at noon. The result is you get the Siderial Time for the moment of the birth. Now you can read from the Tables of Ascendants the particular degree of the Rasi (Sign) that rises at that place.

After getting the figure for the ascendant you will proceed to find out the cusp of the 10th house or the Meridian Cusp (M.C.) which is essential for calculating all the remaining houses or Bhavas. This also can be ascertained from the Table of Ascendants instead of going into the various calculations. Then you have to find out the planets or the Grahasphutas for the time of the birth. For this purpose we can utilise the Lahiri's Indian Ephemeris of that particular year wherein the Nirayana lattitudes of the planets are given for 5.30 A.M. for each day. By knowing the movements of the planets time correction can be given to get at the correct time positions. Similarly calculation of *Bhavas* can also be done by working out the *Sandhis* of various houses. But I do want to go into the details of this as it needs some mathematical background etc. and the common man need not be burdened with this. After getting the chart one can prepare its navamsa chart also as explained in the previous pages. An example chart is given herewith for easy understanding:

Name: Ch. Srinivasa Rao

Date of Birth: 21-6-1967

Time of Birth: 5.50 A.M.

Place of Birth: Chirala, Prakasma Dt., A.P.

	10	11	12	1				
9	Saturn (18.05)	Rahu (11.56)		L (8.03) Sun (6.43) Mercury (28.11)				Mercury
		RASI		Jupiter (11.41) Venus (21.45)	2		Navamsa	Rahu
8					3	Venus Ketu		Mars (R)
7		Moon (19.45)	Ketu (11.56)	R Mars (25.25)		L Moon Saturn Sun	Jupiter	
		6	5	4				

5.50 a.m.   Chirala: 15.50:80.25
                      m   s
                   -8.32 + .01

Please note that always Lagna is the Ist house and from there the other houses are marked. In the given example the Lagna (L) is Mithuna and the Rasi is Vrischika i.e. where the Moon is posted.

At this juncture it becomes necessary to two upagrahas or minor planets to be mentioned that is Gulika and Mandi and these are said to be the sons of Saturn. Some do not make any distinction between the both and there are some who do not recognise these two. So it is better we know this much about them at this stage, and not to bother further.

Each of the 12 houses represent a number of things which you should know. But it is enough we know the important thing represented by them which are as follows:

1st House: This is also called Lagna and it denotes complexion, caste, physical appearance, mental characteristics, nature of birth, fame and defame, success etc., general health, childhood and personality.

2nd House: Signifies family, speech, vision and financial prosperity, in short the second house largely but not exclusively indicates wealth.

3rd House: Rules brothers, sisters and relatives in general. It has governance over courage. It is concerned with throat, ears and father's death. In respect to brothers and sisters, the reference is generally to younger ones i.e. those born after the native.

4th House: This has reference to mother, immovable properties, education, vehicles and general happiness.

5th House: Refers to children, emotions and feelings, faith in God and Poorvapunya. To a certain extent it is also concerned with speculative tendencies.

6th House: Signifies accidents, diseases, enemies, mental affliction, mother's brother and misfortunes.

7th House: Mainly refers to marriage, wife or husband and marital happiness.

8th House: Deals with longevity, legacies, gifts and

unearned wealth, nature of death, disgrace, degradation and details pertaining to death.

9th House: Signifies father, righteousness, preceptor, grand children, intution, religion, sympathy, fame, charities, leadership, long-jouneys and communication with spirits. Is primarily concerned with father and long distance travel. (Foreign also).

10th House: Refers to occupations, profession, temporal honours, foreign travels, self-respect, knowledge and dignity and means of livelihood.

11th House: Refers to gains, elder brother, friends, acquisitions, freedom from misery and happy tidings. To some extent the eleventh house also concerns marriage.

12th House: Signifies losses, extravagance, expenditure, confiscation, sayana-sukha (pleasures of the couch or bed-comforts), left eye, feet, incarceration, divine knowledge and piety and final emancipation (Moksha).

4. Planetary Strength

Now we shall know about the strength of the planets. A planet which owns both Kendra and a Kona house is called Yogakaraka bestower of benefits - his aspect cannot be harmful despite his malefic nature. Similarly planets that occupy constellations that are 3rd, 5th or 7th counted from that of the ascendant or the Moon yield untoward results or effects. You may bear in mind that planets do not exercise their aspects in the Navamsa chart as they do in the Rasi chart.

Now in the chart the houses have different names: The 1st, 4th, 7th and 10th are termed Kendras or Angles; the 5th and 9th are called Trikonas or Trines; the 2nd, 5th, 8th and 11th are called panaparas; and the 3rd, 6th, 9th and 12th are termed Apoklima. The 3rd, 6th, 10th and 11th are called Upachayas or houses of progress. Another way of looking at this is: Mercury and Jupiter are always strong in the lagna, whatever be the Rasi: The Sun and Mars in the 10th; the Moon and Venus in the 4th house, and Saturn in the 7th. This is called as **Digbala** or Directional strength. As you know the lagna represents the East, the 4th North, 7th West and 10th South. The four houses mentioned here happen to be the Kendras or Angular Houses. All planets are strong in Kendras, especially benefics are strong there; they are moderately strong in Panapara Houses; and weak in Apoklimas. It is to be remembered that for malefics ownership of Kendras is very good, while for benefics occupation of Kendra is beneficial.

Planets have a sixfold strength: Kalaja or one born of the time (Temporal), Chesta (motional), Ucha or one derived from the exaltation position, Dik (Directional), Ayna or one derived from its declination, and Sthana

(Positional). Mars, Moon and the Venus are strong at night. The benefics are powerful in the bright fortnight and the malefics in the dark fortnight. Mercury is strong always. The rest are strong during the day. According to Horasastra even Saturn is strong at night. The strength of the planets is measured in Rupas.

The Sun gets the Chestabala in his northerly direction the Moon gets it when she is full; and others get it when they are retrograde. In planetary war (Grahayuddha)—when two planets are positional in the same degree, they are said to be at War and that planet which is to the North of the others is called the Victorious one (of course there are many varieties of victories). The victorious planet as well as those that possess plenty of brilliant rays also get this Chestabala.

Planets get their Ucchabala of 1 Rupa when they are in their highest exaltation.

The Ayanabla is got by Mercury, Saturn and Moon when they are in their southerly course and the rest in their northerly course. Now the last or sixth is the Sthanabala or positional strength. Consideration of a planet's position in exaltation own house, friendly house etc., is the basis of this positional strength. Planets posted in kendras get one Rupa as their strength those in panaparas half Rupa, and those in Apoklima one fourth Rupa. A planet in his own Navamsa is said to be strong in Sthana. A planet in exaltation gets 1 Rupa, in Mulatrikona, ½ in his own house, in a friend's house and nil in enemy's house, depression and combustion. There is another kind of bala: A hermaphrodite (eunuch) planet is strong in the middle of the Rasi, a male planet in its initial part, and a female planet at its end. Similarly among the planets Mars is naturally twice as strong as Saturn, Mercury is 4 times as strong as Mars, Jupiter 8 times as Mercury, Venus 8 times as Jupiter, and Moon sixteen times as Venus, and Sun twice as the Moon, lastly Rahu is twice as strong as the Sun. So now the strength of the luminaries is very important for the well-being of the Native. A planet though otherwise strong will spoil the Rasi/Bhava it occupies and owns, if it is eclipsed. Even if such a planet should form any Yoga, it would not be of much value. If benefic planets are stronger than malefics, the native will become fortunate, attractive, brave and brilliant. If contrary is the case, sinful, cruel, and foolish fellows are born. Planets are said to be badly positioned when they are eclipsed, debilitated (nicha) in Rasi or Navamsa, positioned in the sign of enemy, in the 6th, 8th or 12th house from Lagna. In other positions they are said to be well-placed. Generally the planets are strong in their exaltation; the Moon is strong when she has Pakshabala; and the Sun is strong when he has Digbala in full i.e. in the 10th house from the Lagna which is also known as the Meridian.

Planets to be positioned in Kendras is a matter of considerable strength for the planets. Among the 4 kendras the Lagna-kendra is the strongest, next in importance is the 7th, next to that is the 10th and last is the 4th which is called as Patala. There are two kinds of friendships etc. existing amongst the planets, natural and temporary. Of these the former is more powerful and lasting. Although Venus is 8 times as strong as Jupiter, still Jupiter being the preceptor of the Gods and philosophical in nature has no parallel in conferring good results on Humanity. He is therefore, very powerful in warding off evil influences and conferring all sorts of benefits. Venus has only half the strength of Jupiter in these matters, while Mercury only of Jupiter power. However, the strength of the Moon is the primary cause of that of all the planets. So, if Moon is weak in a horoscope, much of its power is lost.

There is another source of strength: A planet in exaltation is the first, one in the Mulatrikona is the second; one in his own house is the third; one in a friend's house is the fourth; one in the varga of a benefic planet is the fifth, one with a mass of brilliant rays sixth; one defeated in a planetary war (Garhayuddha) the 7th; one positioned in the Varga (Rasi, Hora etc.,) of a malefic the 8th; one in an enemy's house the 9th; one in debilitation the 10th and lastly an eclipsed one is the 11th. The good effect of a planet in the

Pardiptavasta will be full and in the last nil. In the others it is proportional to the place between the two extremes.

It is very essential for a long and happy life to have the Lagna and the Moon as well as their lords to be strong. What is meant by the Lord of the Moon? It is the lord of the house occupied by her. There is another way of finding out the age of the planets. A planet occupying its own or friendly house is said to be in boyhood; one in the Mulatrikona, in youth; in Exaltation, in the position of a prince of yuvaraja; in Inimical house, in old age and in Debilitation, in death.

Before proceeding further let us understand the Ududasa system which will also stand you in good stead in determining the span of life. Ancients have declared that the span of human life is 120 years. This period is distributed among 9 planets thus—The Sun's Dasa coming first in this scheme is for 6 years, the next Moon for 10 years, then of Mars for 7 years, then of Rahu for 18 years, then of Jupiter is for 16 years, then of Saturn for 19 years, then of Mercury for 17 years, then of Ketu for 7 years and lastly Venus for 20 years. Though the Dasa-order is this, do not think that all persons begin with the Sun's dasa or major period. As this is called Ududasa—Udu means star the major period is found out from the star tenented by the Moon at the time of birth. The following table will show the stars which produce the Dasas of the different planets—

Sun—Krittika, Uttaraphalguni and Uttarashada.

Moon—Rohini, Hasta and Sravana.

Mars—Mrigasira, Chitta and Dhanista.

Rahu—Aridra, Swathi and Satabhisham.

Jupiter—Punarvasu, Visakha and Purvabhadra.

Saturn—Pushyami, Anuradha, and Uttarabhadra.

Mercury—Aslesha, Jyesta, and Revathi.

Ketu—Magha, Mula and Aswini.

Venus—Purvaphalguni, Purvasada and Bharani.

Now we have to find out what portion of a particular Dasa is already over in the state of pregnancy and what portion of it still remains at birth. The most popular method of calculating this is the following: find out from a good Panchanga (Almanac) the total duration of the particular star of birth, as well as the part that has already elapsed at the time of birth. Then you can easily find out the remaining part of the star. You know for the full star the number of years allotted. Let X be the total duration of the Nakshatra in Ghatis, Y be the unexpired portion of that star in Ghatis and Z be the number of years allotted to that star. Then the balance of the Dasa in stars will be equal to $Y/X \times Z$. Any fraction of a year is to be multiplied by 12 and divided by the same denominator. This will give you the months. If any fraction of a month remains, it should be multiplied by 30 and divided as before. This will give you the days. But readymade tables are available with the Ephemeris of each year. From that table the figure could be ascertained without going into the calculations. Hence, the readers can refer to the tables and get the figures and proceed further.

5. Span of Life

Sages have declared that it is not possible to determine the span of life of a human being until he/she is 12 years of age. He may die within four years owing to the previous sins of his mother, or within 8 years on account of the sins of his father and lastly by his own sins. The cause of his death during this period is called Balarista. To ward off this evil influence people are advised to perform propitiatory Homas on the day of the child's Janmanakshatra and to take proper medical advice also. According to another view, the Balarista period lasts for only 8 years. There is another Arista called Yogarista, evil planetary configurations which might cause death before the age of 20 years. If the span extends beyond 20 but not 32, it is termed short life or Alpayu; if the life extends upto 70, it is Madhyayu or moderate span; and beyond that it is full. Still, the human span of 100 years being divided into 3 equal parts would give us the three types of life.

There are some Yogas or planetary configurations which lead to early death of the native. If the Ascendant at birth is the very end of a Sign which is aspected or occupied by malefics, immediate death is possible. If it is at a Gandanta, the father, mother or the child might quit the world. Should the child survive, it would become as great as a King. If the birth is any one of the four kinds of Sandhis which receive the aspect of malefics or cojoined with them, early death is predicted. Though you may be sure of the coming end, you should not utter an inauspicious word. Your business is to say that there are many evil influences which should be warded off by means of proper worship, prayers etc. of the planets and their deities presiding over them. The end aim of Astrology is not merely to predict the coming events but to strengthen the devotion to God and thus lead them to the path of spirituality culminating in self-realisation. The astrologer should be a practical philosopher. There are some yogas for early death. They are as follow:

(1) If the lord of lagna and the benefics are all placed in Apoklimas houses i.e. 3,6,9 and 12.

(2) If the malefics and lord of the 8th house occupy Kendras.

(3) If the lords of Lagna and the 8th are inimical to each other or if the lords of the Chandra-lagna and of the 8th therefore are inimical to each other or if the Sun and the Lagna-lord are mutual enemies. Please bear in mind that these are the general rules which may be rendered inoperative on account of other powerful factors such as the position of strong Jupiter in the Ascendant.

The following yogas are leading to long and medium lease of life—benefics and lord of Lagna should be in Kendras. The same being in panapara houses (2, 5, 8, 11) cause medium life. If malefics and the lord of the 8th house occupy Apoklima and Panapara Houses, long and medium life respectively are caused. If the three pairs of planets are friendly, long life is the result, If they are neutral medium life. If the lord being very strong is posted in a Kendra and is aspected by benefics and not all by malefics, the person is blessed with long life, virtue and prosperity. A strong Jupiter in the Lagna can singly ward off a hundred evil yogas. Similarly the presence of the Sun— for day-birth and the Moon for night-birth in the 11th Bhava from the lagna has the power of warding off a crore of Doshas according to Sage Garga.

I would like to clarify that the year 32 in person's life is critical. It is called Dwatrimsadayoga. If this coincides with any Dasa-sandhi or other bad period, the native may die, provided there are yogas for short life. This is the reason for the statement that it is a bad time for a person when Saturn in his transit passes through the position occupied by him at birth. Now we must know as to how long do the planets stay in a house during their transit. The Sun generally takes one month, the Moon two days and a quarter. Mars two months, Mercury one month, Jupiter one year, Venus one month, Saturn two years and half and Rahu-Ketu one year and six months. According to this measure Saturn makes one complete circuit in 30 years. In the case of short life death takes place in the first round of the Saturn, of medium life in the second round, and of long life in the third. Now you must be anxious to know when the death takes place exactly. The following is the method for finding this: Add up the longitudes of the Sun, Moon, Jupiter and Saturn at birth. When saturn passes through the positions indicated by this sum in one of his rounds, death is likely.

Longevity (length of life) can be divided into 4 groups (1) Balarista or Early death—up to 8 years, (2) Alapayu or Short life—8 years to 32 years, (3) Madhyayu or Medium life—32 to 75 years. (4) Purnayu or Full Life—75 years to 120 years. It is enough if we know this much about the span of life. There is a generalised statement to know the different spans of life and the same is given below so that by a glance at the statement, one can know the span of life of an individual:

Longevity Chart

Long Life (75 to 120 yr.)	Medium Life (32 to 75 yr.)	Short Life (8 to 32 yr.)
1. Lagna and the 8th lords in moveable signs (Chara Rasis).	1. Lagna lord in moveable and 8th lord in fixed.	1. Lagna lord in moveable and 8th lord in common sign.
2. Lagna lord in a fixed sign (sthira) and 8th lord in common sign (Ubhaya)	2. Lagna lord in fixed sign and 8th lord in moveable sign.	2. Lagna lord in fixed and 8th lord in fixed.
3. Lagna lord in common sign (Ubhaya) and 8th lord in fixed sign (Sthira).	3. Lagna lord in common and 8th lord in common sign.	3. Lagna lord in common and 8th lord in moveable sign.

6. Rasi Effects

Each Zodiac sign has certain qualities. Let us see the general character of the people born under these various Zodiac divisions.

Aries — Mesha

People born under this are of an independent view. They are educated, they love science and philosophy. They follow certain good principles in life. They are quick in thought. The lord of the house is Mars which stands for bravery. They are not bulky but strong. They can work for several hours to solve a problem. The lord of 5th and 9th (Sun and Jupiter) are good. The lords of 3, 6, 11, (Mercury Saturn) do not give good results.

Taurus — Vrishabha

This is the bull. They are not very tall when compared to others. Mathematics appeal to this class than others. Literary taste in early life can be seen. They prefer business to regular job. Their memory is generally strong and sharp. When Mercury is well placed, they become great writers. Since they are quick in thought and actions certain extent of wrong calculations of events are also likely. When they are angry they get out of control. The lords of 5, 9 (Mercury, Saturn) are good. The lords of 3, 6, 11 (Moon, Venus Jupiter) are bad. There is a peculiarity in this. Venus as lord of the house is not benefic.

Gemini — Mithuna

They are rarely idle. They have mechanical brain. They can learn many things in life. In every field they have knowledge. Mercury is a nervous planet. This moves quickly and the nature is the same in the family life also. They get excited quickly. Restriction in indulgence is quite needed otherwise they may suffer from nervousness to a great extent. Operations or fire accidents are also likely. Venus and Saturn are good. Sun, Mars, Jupiter are unfavourable.

Cancer — Kataka

This class is more intelligent. They develop respect for others. They have deep attachment for family and children. They have justice in their talk. Though they are sympathetic they are talkative. Generally they are successful in life. Mars and Jupiter are favourable; Mercury, Venus are unfavourable. Though Jupiter is the 6th lord it is not unfavourable. Mars-Jupiter combination is very good. When Jupiter is in 6th he becomes only bad and when it is in the 9th he happens to be good.

Leo — Simha

This indicates lion. Their physical appearance is also somewhat like lion with broad chest and majestic look. Ambition is inborn nature. They love fine arts. They are religious minded. They respect old ways and traditions. They are very ideal with the result that they never adapt to circumstances or environments in life. This is the reason for their fight for success. Jupiter and Mars are favourable whereas Venus, Mercury and Saturn are not favourable.

Virgo — Kanya

Generally this class is not very beautiful. They are carried away by emotions and do things by impulse. Music appeals to this class more than others. Venus is the lord of 2nd and hence all kinds of arts appeal. They can become efficient also. Saturn becomes the lord of the 5th and 6th and hence his position and aspect is very important point. Venus and Mercury are good. Nervous troubles and stomach troubles are often seen.

Libra — Tula

A balanced man physically and mentally. They have power of observation and reason out men and matters. They do reform society and remove evils in society. They are attached to home and surroundings. They never care for others or their say. They become famous. Often they exhibit certain amount of intution faculty. Saturn confers yoga. Mercury, Saturn in favourable houses do good and Moon-Mercury combination is very good.

Scorpio — Vrischika

This is another masculine sign. They are unsteady and get excited easily. Martial traits are seen even in ladies. Music appeals to them and when learnt regularly they can become proficient. They are hot. In matters of health some get venereal diseases also. As jupiter being the 2nd and 5th they learn well. Jupiter, Moon and Sun are good. Mercury and venus are bad. 2, 5, 9, 10 are controlled by Jupiter, Moon and Sun. When they are well placed great results can be expected.

Sagittarius — Dhanus

This class as Jupiter (Guru) indicates following orthodox principles. They like occult subjects. By nature they are God fearing. They have fine manners. They exercise control over emotions. Mars with combination of Sun give very excellent result.

Capricorn — Makara

People of this class are the tallest of all the classes. They rarely complain and have adaptability to any environment.

Though they always wish to be economical they are not so practically. They are sympathetic to fellowmen. When provoked they become vindictive also. Venus is the powerful planet that can do much help. When there is a combination of Mercury and Venus in favourable house, better results are seen. Bile and knee joints give trouble.

Aquarius — Kumbha

This is the most difficult sign to be understood. Great people are born under this sign. Intelligence is inborn in them. They have a large circle of friends. They get angry quickly and also get cooled easily. Because they are shy and moody, most of them do not shine well. They learn occult sciences. They have great attachment to home and family as Venus plays a prominent role.

Pisces — Meena

These people are reserved in temperament. By nature they are God fearing. They respect friendship. They have liking for old things like coins etc. Though they appear as independent, in reality it is seldom. Mars is favourable and when there is Moon, Mars, Jupiter combination it is very good.

Effects of planets occupying exaltation, own houses friendly etc. Exaltation: The subject is likely to become a big landlord or king, and being possessed of immense wealth. He will be endowed with excellent virtues, victorious everywhere, famous, charitable, courageous, clever and diplomatic.

Own house: The person concerned will have during the Dasa of that planet power and pelf, he will stay in his own house permanently, will acquire new house and fertile lands, receive respect from the people and recover all lost articles.

Friendly house: He will achieve his objects with the help of friends, make new friends, have the good fortune of the company of wife and sons. He will enjoy wealth and corn, will be charitable and friend of all and enemy to none.

Inimical house: He becomes lowly, eats others' food, stays in others' houses, becomes indigent, is troubled always by rivals and foes, and even a friend turns out to be an inveterate enemy.

Debilitation: He will have a fall from his position, experience poverty, contraction of debts and indulgence in wicked acts. He will make friends with igonable, be in servitude, will walk long distances and do unprofitable tasks. He will reside in unhealthy places.

Combustion: He may quit the world in the period of the concerned planet, will be deprived of his wealth, wife and children. He will quarrel for nothing, he will be the object of scandal, humiliation and defeat.

A planet posted in a neutral house will enable one to maintain his statusquo. The effects of Vargottamamsa—a planet occupying the same Rasi both in Rasi and Navamsa charts—are equal to those of one in own house. You may be interested to know what will be the effect of debilitated planets both in Rasi and Amsa e.g. Venus in the last Navamsa of Virgo. Though you may technically call it a case of Vargottamamsa, yet in fact it is extremely bad.

7. On Bhavas

Bhava-Karakas: We are aware of the names of the twelve Bhavas beginning with Tanu-Body. Each of these Bhavas has one or more Karakas or Significators who are permanent presidents. They are in order (1) the Sun, (2) Jupiter, (3) Mars, (4) The Moon and Mercury, (5) Jupiter, (6) Saturn and Mars, (7) Venus, (8) Saturn, (9) the Sun and Jupiter (10) the Sun, Mercury, Jupiter and Saturn, (11) Jupiter, and (12) Saturn. From this one can see that the Sun has three portfolios, of the 1st, 9th and 10th. The moon and Venus have only one each viz. 4th and 7th respectively. Mars has two, the 3rd and the 6th. Mercury too has two viz. the 4th and 10th. Jupiter has five and Saturn four. From this it would be seen that Jupiter and Saturn hold extraordinary positions in the life of human beings.

Please remember that benefics in auspicious Bhavas—those except the Dusthanas, 6, 8, 12—enhance their good effects, while in evil houses they tone down their bad effects. Similarly malefics in good houses, spoil their good effects, except when they are owners of such houses, and enhance the bad effects of the evil houses they are in. In principle karakas should not occupy the particular bhava. Jupiter though karaka for five Bhavas, 2, 5, 9, 10 and 11 yet he is bad only for the 5th Bhava i.e. issue, if he is posted in that Bhava. When you want to know all about a Bhava, consider that as the starting point i.e. Lagna and take next house therefrom as its house of wealth or family. For example if you want to know all the details about a subject's father, take the 9th house as the Lagna and proceed further. The 9th house from this new lagna would give you an idea about subject's paternal grandfather. Similary take the 4th house in the case of the mother. The strength of the Bhava, its Karaka and lord, as well as aspects etc. should be borne in mind while assessing the worth of the Bhava. In this connection, there are relationships or Sambandha among the planets in a chart. There are five kinds of relationship viz: (1) exchange of positions between two planets or what is known as planets in mutual reception, (2) conjunction of the two, (3) mutual aspect, (4) to be in Mutual Kendras or quadrants, and (5) to be in mutual konas or trines. This much of knowledge will help to ascertain if the lords of the Karakas of a Bhava are in good or bad relationship between themselves. For example, it is bad for the lord of the Bhava to be posted in a Dusthana, 6, 8, 12 from that Bhava.

Now I should like to give the effects of the presence of the planets in the different Bhavas.

Sun

1st House

When Sun in lagna (1st house) gets a favourable aspect, this position indicates sharp intelligence. As the Sun is a hot planet, the constitution also is very hot. Sun stands for Satwa Guna and hence generally this person will have more purity of mind. There will be good moral standard.

2nd House

This indicates good learning. Education in science can be expected. They are generous. Their talk reflect some brilliance of their learning.

3rd House

This indicates wealthy conditions and bravery. They have good taste for art.

4th House

This is Mathrusthana and Sun in this position is not good for mother. There will be constant hindrances in life. If favourable planets aspect this house or when 4th house happens to be that of Sun then the health of mother will not be affected.

5th House

This is not a favourable place either for children or father. Mental worry is the result.

6th House

The native will be very brave in life. They can plan matters well. Wealthy condition can be expected. Victory over enemies can also be earned. Good prospect in art line is also seen.

7th House

This is very unfavourable position. Unless benefic planets aspect, early marriage is not seen. This gives loose morals.

8th House

Long life is indicated but the constitution will be weak. If favourable planet aspect this position, some good results can be achieved. However, the eyesight will be affected.

9th House

Astronomy suits this class. There will be higher studies. They are Godly and self supporting. Favourable results to father are seen. All kinds of art lines appeal to them. They will be charitable.

10th House

This is a very favourable position. High position in Govt. is often seen. One can become efficient in sciences. As they are very clever, they earn well. They will have dutiful sons. Political career is also very likely.

11th House

Early success, status in society are indicated. They have certain set principles in life. They get Royal Honour. They enjoy life well.

12th House

This is a very bad position. Moral standard is not seen. Giving up harsh traits in nature. This can confirm Atma Gyana also when there is effort in this course.

Moon

1st House

When this is her own house and gets favourable aspect the native will be in art lines, if otherwise there is no fixity in life. There will be more struggles.

2nd House

Royal honour is indicated. They will be wealthy. As the moon is having bright and dark period there will be breaks in education. As moon is described silvery in speech, the speech will be quite attractive.

3rd House

This is an unfavourable position. There will be some kind of ailment in the body almost always. A female planet in Bhrathrusthana indicates more sisters.

4th House

This is Mathrusthana and Karaka in that house indicates property from mother side. These people will be successful in life. If unfavourable planets aspect this, the health of the mother will be affected.

5th House

This is an interesting position in a way. The wife will be fair and more daughters can be seen as female planet in Putrasthana. Wealth through cattle is indicated. There will be constant hindrances in education. If aspected by benefics the position will improve.

6th House

Moral standard is very low. Connection with widows, stealing habit, drinking habit etc. are indicated.

7th House

A good family life is seen. Health of the mother will be affected. The man will be energetic. Wealth or position through wife is indicated. The position of Moon in this, in the case of ladies will give a devoted husband but one who changes his ideas and doubts.

8th House

This is a very bad position. If there is any aspect by benefic there will be some relief. If there is no such aspect the life will be in danger.

9th House

They are intelligent and well educated. They read more and more. They are charitable. They are fond of travel. Religion and devotion to God is inborn. This is a favourable position; if there is aspect of benefics great gains by sudden means can be expected.

10th House

Moon is powerful in this position. Good health, landed properties, income through water sources, good wife etc. will be the result.

11th House

They enjoy high status in society, success in life and help from fair sex are indicated. There is interest in in art. They become influential.

12th House

This is an unfavourable position. Gain in unlawful paths, solitude etc. will be the result.

Mars

1st House

The constitution is hot as indicated by the Mars, if this happens to be his own house with the aspect of benefics, then Mars will do all good things. Otherwise constant fight will be the outcome.

2nd House

This is not a good house. They will quarrel always as they get angry quickly.

3rd House

As indicator of brothers and 3rd place is Bhatrusthana, few brothers are indicated. Help through brothers are indicated. There will not be high moral standards, however.

4th House

This gives conveniences and comforts but very unhappy family life. Mother's health will be affected. If this happens to be his own house and wherein aspect be benefic, good results are expected.

5th House

This is a bad place. This indicates putra dosham. Mind will be diverted on wrong path. There may not be children or children may not be useful.

6th House

The man will be courageous. Enemies will be afraid of him. His health will be moderate. Some status in political line is indicated, 6th is otherwise 9th place when counted from his 10th place. Hence, Mars has some power in this place.

7th House

This is a bad position. Late marriage is likely. This should have aspect by benefic for good results. Maternal property is obtained. The man will be intelligent.

8th House

This is another bad position for Mars. If there is no favourable aspect this may give short life to wife, eye defect, loose morals etc.

9th House

This is also a bad position. Sickness to father is indicated. Stubborn nature is seen. Business or trade overseas is also likely.

10th House

This is a good position. One will be self made. He will be energetic and active. Landed properties are expected. There will be happiness in life. As lord of 5th if he is in 10th, very good results can be seen. For Cancer the sign Scorpio is 5th and when Mars is in Aries which is 10th to Cancer, very great results are achieved.

11th House

The native will be highly learned. He will possess helping mind. Cordial relation among his brothers is seen. They will be influential. Royal honour can be expected.

12th House

This is a very bad place. Delay in marriage. Constant difficulties and unsuccessful career are the results.

Mercury

1st House

This gives vast learning. There is interest in the study of occult sciences. This gives reputation.

2nd House

Religion and philosophy appeal to this class. They are fluent speakers. They will have good wife and helping relations. They are clever, hence they earn well.

3rd House

This is a favourable position with regard to brothers. Certain amount of miserliness with stubborn nature and hard heartedness are also seen.

4th House

This position is good for mothers. Ancestral property, income through literary activities are seen. Agriculture appeals more.

5th House

They become learned and get respect from wealthy persons. They are good administrators. This is a bad position for children or health of parents or maternal relations.

6th House

This is not a good place for Mercury. This will give break in education. There will be vanity. There may not be enemies in life. Loss is indicated.

7th House

Success in art, ill health to mother, marriage at an early age are all indicated. They are God fearing. They have taste for learning occult sciences.

8th House

Long life is indicated. They will be respected. They will possess landed property. They save for rainy days of life.

9th House

This is a very good position. The man will have many children. He will be philosophical. He will be having great taste for literature and music. He will become popular and influential.

10th House

This is an interesting and good place. They become intelligent and earn easily. They are fortunate in life. There will be many enjoyments in life. They command good respect in society. They have great devotion to God. They are business minded.

11th House

Astrology or Mathematics appeals to this class. The health will be moderately good. As businessmen they earn well. They will have large circle of friends.

12th House

They become passionate. There may not be many

issues but they will be worried always. They will be philosophical.

Jupiter

1st House

This is a good place. His aspect falls on 5th and 9th places with majestic look, they are good in appearance. They become learned. They get respect and Royal honour. They are leaders also. They are endowed with good children.

2nd House

They are fluent and good speakers with refined manners. They get adjusting partner. There is humour in their talk. They are fortunate and have number of friends.

3rd House

This confers many brothers. They develop devotion to family. Though there is a taste for literature, agriculture appeals more.

4th House

A kendra position. Jupiter is not so advantageous. With good education there will be contentment in life. This is a good position as Matrusthana.

5th House

This can give ability. This is putrasthana. There is a saying that jupiter spoils the house in which he is situated but elevates the house which he aspects. As a karaka for putra his position here may not give many children. As purvapunyasthana indicates intelligence and devotion.

6th House

They are unsuccessful though intelligent. There may not be any enemies.

7th House

One can be helped by the partner. There is speculative

tendency. Agriculture appeals more, when jupiter is in 7th kendra. Dosha comes, known as kendrathipathya dosham.

8th House

This is not a good place. Long life is seen. Unclean habits and unhappiness are seen.

9th House

Devotion to religion and God fearing nature are inborn. With certain good principles they become learned and cultured. They give plenty of wealth to charities or institutions.

10th House

Agriculture appeals more. The profession will meet constant hindrances. Some status in society is obtained.

11th House

Being self made they become wealthy. They do noble deeds. They are charitable minded. They excercise sufficient influence in society

12th House

This is a bad position. They become sinful, unless it is his own house or has good aspects, this is not good. Some mantra upadesa is likely.

Note: The position of jupiter plays a vital role in life. It is indeed fortunate to have jupiter in favourable position or to have his aspect in favourable bhavas or born in a Lagna to which he is a yogakaraka.

Venus

1st House

This is a good position. They become learned and have great taste for music. With good health long life is seen, sudden wealth is also seen. They are fortunate.

2nd House

A happy family life with many relations are seen. A beautiful life-partner is obtained. Property acquisition is likely.

3rd House

This position is good for brothers. The life will not be very smooth. The native will have evil ideas.

4th House

This is also a favourable position. Education, vehicles, property, good health of mother are all indicated. 4th place Venus is good.

5th House

As a natural enemy for jupiter putrakaraka, in his 5th house karakathava venus is bad. This gives some putra dosha also. Mother's health will be affected. There will be more daughters than sons. High education and political success are expected.

6th House

There will be worries from enemies. Loose habits are likely. Health will be affected unless the individual is careful. He will have ailment in generative organs.

7th House

This is a very bad position for Venus. As a karaka for family in this sthana, he does not confer family happiness. Though one may become wealthy, his mind will run on wrong path.

8th House

Mother's health will be affected. Bad society and evil habits are likely.

9th House

This confers high learning and respect in society. They are generous and successful in life. But they are not free from selfishness.

10th House
They develop respect for Divine persons and also great devotion to God. The education is often broken. To some extent, political success is seen.

11th House
This is favourable position. They are brave and courageous. They can get high education. They are attracted by fair sex. They become very popular in society.

12th House
This is not an advantageous position for ladies. At a later stage Bhakti (devotion to god) will dawn. In the early stages the mind is preoccupied with evil thoughts.

Saturn

1st House
Evil thoughts, evil ways, misery, perversity of mind are the outcome. Lagna, aspects on lagna have to be considered.

2nd House
This is a very bad place for wife and family. The speech will be harsh.

3rd House
This is a bad position for brothers. Though this position can confer intelligence and wealth, the life will be adventurous. Agriculture appeals more.

4th House
This is another unfavourable position for mother and when moon is also in this place, it is very bad. There will be constant problems in the career.

5th House
Children will be sickly. In some cases there will be no children. Education will suffer at many stages. There will be more vices.

6th House

This will increase debts and diseases. Pain in joints or bile trouble are often noticed.

7th House
Evil mind, bad company, very late marriage are the outcome.

8th House
Long life is expected. Ayushkaraka in Ayushthana is good to confer long life. Very poor condition of life is also there.

9th House
The native will suffer due to poverty. No help from any body can be expected.

10th House
This is moderately good. Patient study of higher mathematics or sciences is noticed. The person shall possess many vehicles. The native is religious minded.

11th House
There will be wealth and success. Success in political activities are also likely. They can exercise great influence on society.

12th House
There will be a device to study occult sciences. Sickness with poverty will prevail. If there is any aspect of benefics, certain amount of relief can be seen.

Saturn in any house (except 10-11), cannot confer anything great. But persons born in Taurus or Libra are saved. Others are his victims. Nobody can completely avoid his play in life since saturn has to be in any one of the 12 houses. Right thinking, going on the right path, doing charity will minimise the punishment of Saturn.

Rahu and Ketu

They have no ownership over any house. They take the role of the house in which they are placed and the combinations with which they are seen, or the aspects they get decide their course. They can do good or bad of the house in which they are placed to a greater degree. However the behaviour of these two are given below:

Rahu

1st House

Obliging, sympathetic, abortion, courageous, sickly wife or husband.

2nd House

Poor and more than one wife if afflicted, dark complexion, diseased face, peevish, luxurious habits.

3rd House

Few children, wealthy, bold, adventurous, courageous, good gymnast, many relations.

4th House

Liaison with women of easy virtue, subordinate, proficient in European languages.

5th House

Childless, flatulent, tyrranical, polite, narrow minded and hard-headed.

6th House

Enjoyment, venereal complaints, no enemies, many cousins.

7th House

Wife suffering from menstural disorders, widow or divorcee connection, diabetes, luxurious food, unhappy.

8th House

Vicious, degraded, quarrelsome, narrow minded, immoral, adulterous.

9th House
A puppet in the hands of his wife, impolite, uncharitable, emaciated waist, loose morals.

10th House
Intimacy with widows, taste in poetry and literature, good artist, traveller, learned.

11th House
Wealthy, influential among lower castes, many children, good agriculturist.

12th House
Deformed, few children, defective sight, very many losses, saintly.

Ketu

1st House
Emaciated figure, weak constitution, much perspiration, weak-hearted, slender, piles, sexual indulgence, diplomatic.

2nd House
Bad speaker, quiet, quick in perception, peevish, hard-hearted, thrifty and economical.

3rd House
Adventurous, strong, artistic, wealthy, popular.

4th House
Quarrelsome, licentious, weak, fear of poisons.

5th House
Liberal, loss of children, sinful, immoral if afflicted.

6th House
Fond of adultery, good conversationist, licentious, venereal complaints learned.

7th House

Passionate, sinful, connections with widows, sickly wife.

8th House

Senseless, obscure, dull, sanguine complexion, piles and similar troubles.

9th House

Short sighted, sinful, untruthful, thrifty, many children, good wife.

10th House

Fertile brain, happy, religious, pilgrimages to sacred rivers and places, fond of scriptures.

11th House

Humorous, witty, licentious, intelligent, wealthy.

12th House

Capricious, unsettled mind, foreign residence, attracted to servile classes, much travelling, licentious, spiritual knowledge.

8. Planets and Signs

We have seen the results of the planets in various bhavas. A particular bhava may be any sign—either own house or Neecha position and more than one planet may also be combined. The significance of each planet as lord of a particular Bhava in a particular sign to be well understood.

For example take Scorpio as lagna. The Lord of 10th is Sun. If he is in cancer, he is in the 9th house, a watery sign. A fiery planet in a watery sign. Like this all other signs may be seen. So, let us see some more details.

Sun

In Aries: He is exalted here. The nature of the Sun is light and brilliant. Hence, it makes the native ambitious and intelligent. This gives good personality.

In Taurus: This is an evil house for Sun. This is the natural 10th house from his own house Simha. This can give a comfortbale home.

In Gemini: One can become learned and wealthy.

In Cancer: A hot planet in a watery sign. On a rainy day sun is absent. In the same way, the native becomes sickly and sorrowful. This is a bad sign for Sun.

In Leo: Strong in nature with hard-heartedness, one becomes well known for his brilliance.

In Virgo: Learning, memory power, religiousness are indicated.

In Libra: Sun is Neecha. One becomes wicked with loose moral standard.

In Scorpio: Though one is brave and stubborn, he is likely to be carried away by impulsiveness.

In Sagittarius: Religiousness from early age, wealth, popularity are obtained.

In Capricorn: He is an enemy for this sign. Unhappiness and ignorance are the outcome.

In Aquarius: He is not powerful in this sign also. Poverty and failure in this sign also. Poverty and failure in attemps are experienced. Some rare talents also exist.

In Pisces: This confers a peaceful, ordinary life.

Moon

In Aries: Though it can confer vast travel (a watery planet in a fiery sign) unsteady mind and subordinate position are the outcome.

In Taurus: It is her exalted position. Capacity to lead popularity, family happiness etc. are the outcome.

In Gemini: Vast learning, cleverness, taste in music and the like are obtained.

In Cancer: Her own house. Mental power, influence, wealth and voyages are obtained. Mind will be inclined towards meditation, yoga etc. in the later stages.

In Leo: This is a friendly sign. Generosity, ambition and boldness etc. are seen. However, the mind feels some unhappiness.

In Virgo: Intelligence, knowledge in occult sciences are seen. The person will have a set of principles. He will be sincere and honest.

In Libra: This makes one intelligent. He becomes religious-minded and has great regard for holy persons.

In Scorpio: This is his Neecha place. Wealthy position combined with mental agitation and unhappiness are obtained. The native becomes hard-hearted also.

In Sagittarius: Happiness at home, literary gift, strong mind etc are obtained.

In Capricorn: Though it can give cleverness, the mind is unsteady with evil thoughts.

In Aquarius: He is emotional with sudden ups and downs in life.

In Pisces: He is learned and has attachment with wife and children. He is more attracted towards meditation and yoga practices in the advanced stage.

Mars

In Aries: It is in his own house. He is rich and possess, capacity to command. He is social in temperament. He is active and powerful. Frankness with liberal views are also there.

In Taurus: He becomes unprincipled and loose in morals. He is rather emotional and rash at times.

In Gemini: His home and children are pleasant. Music appeals to him. There will be pleasantness in talk, though at times he becomes rash.

In Cancer: One travels wide and becomes rich. Agriculture appeals to this class. There may be perversity of views also. This is his neecha house.

In Leo: He develops independant thinking and has great respect for elders. He is miserly and at times extravagant.

In Virgo: His family life is not very pleasant. He has confidence. He has winning manners.

In Libra: He is ambitious. He earns well, he loses his family. Materialistic tendencies increase.

In Scorpio: He is diplomatic and has sharp memory. With aggressiveness he is proud. However, life is beset with hurdles. It is his own house.

In Sagittarius: There may be court troubles and quarrels. But inspite of these one can become a Statesman and famous.

In Capricorn: His exalted house. Wealthy conditions,

high position, very active, influential.

In Aquarius: Impulsiveness, wandering, controversial mind, unhappiness etc. are also seen.

In Pisces: Passion, unclean habits, troubles in love affairs etc. are the result.

Mercury

In Aries: This is not a good place. Rigidity of views, capacity to bear insults by others, bad company.

In Taurus: Large friends among fair sex, many children and immense riches.

In Gemini: Own house. Great taste in art and literature, one is cultured with affable manners.

In Cancer: Unsteadiness, with minimum moral standards, disliked by relations.

In Leo: Carried away by emotions with sharp memory, one becomes a fluent speaker. He earns well.

In Virgo: Astronomy and religion appeals much. There will be writing capacity. Being learned has high imagination. But has no control over his emotions. This is his ucha place.

In Libra: Goes to extremes. Religiousness and materialism exist side by side. He is a good writer.

In Scorpio: Though brave, he is not calculative of events. He becomes selfish. He comes up well but is not able to maintain the standards.

In Sagittarius: He is learned. Has a high place in society. He is very cunning also. He travels wide.

In Capricorn: He can calculate well before spending, but he is unsteady. Hard-heartedness will also be there.

In Aquarius: One becomes a scholar and gets name and fame. The life will also have hurdles often.

In Pisces: His manners are upto the mark. He is more

childish. It is his neecha place.

Jupiter

In Aries: Indicates riches, many children, winning manners, happy family life.

In Taurus: Good family life with good children, fluency in speech, creative ability are the outcome.

In Gemini: Being well read and learned, he becomes brave and rich.

In Cancer: Vast learning. Intelligence, wealthy conditions are seen. It is his ucha house.

In Leo: He is happy. He is very generous and a man of wisdom. He has great liking for literature.

In Virgo: He is fortunate and full of ambition. He gets charming wife. Selfishness is also seen.

In Libra: He is pleasant man with frankness, manners are fine. Comes up to position quickly but retires soon. Earns well.

In Scorpio: Manners are attractive. Appearance is majestic. Gets help from inlaws' house. He is wealthy and learned. He has good qualities. He becomes an author.

In Sagittarius: He is wealthy and learned. He has got good qualities. He has writing capacity. His own home.

In Capricorn: His Neecha house. He becomes unhappy. There is pessimism.

In Aquarius: Vast learning, popularity, humanitarian deeds.

In Pisces: Property, brilliance and wealth are found in this. His own house.

Venus

In Aries: He has unsteady mind. Literature or art or music appeal. However, moral standard is not high.

In Taurus: Own house. He goes on passionate lines,

he is not steady in mind.

In Gemini: As a materialistic be becomes rich. He has vast learning and becomes a fluent speaker. Comes up well in life.

In Cancer: His views are not steady. He has moods often. He is very sensitive to what others say. He is rich.

In Leo: He gets adjusting wife and help through wife. He becomes passionate. Somehow, he saves much.

In Virgo: He is not happy and gets more enemies. But some riches are also ammased. This is venus' neecha house.

In Libra: A happy home and respect in society are likely. There will be capacity to put forth great effort. One will be patient. This is Venus' own house.

In Scorpio: He is more majestic in mental outlook. This is an ambitious sign.

In Sagittarius: He becomes brave. There will be respect in society. He is generally rich.

In Capricorn: He becomes learned. There will be liking for ladies. He is unprincipled, however.

In Aquarius: With affable and pleasing manners he wins others' hearts. He is rich.

In Pisces: He is calm and does not get excited. He becomes learned. He is religious and wealthy. It is his ucha house.

Saturn

In Aries: One becomes very unlucky. There will be yearning for higher standards of life. It is Saturn's neecha house.

In Taurus: He is very successful. Has the capacity to withstand trials. He is very learned.

In Gemini: Miserable condition, many problems in family. High position is also achieved.

In Cancer: Poverty, failure in attempts.

In Leo: Low mind with stubborn nature. Generally not successful. Sometimes one becomes rich suddenly but the downfall is also equally sudden.

In Virgo: With strong brain power one can put forth maximum efforts, political career appeals more to this class.

In Libra: Very fortunate in life. Generous minded. Commands high respect in society. He is rich. This is saturn's ucha house.

In Scorpio: He is brave to tackle any situation in life. Sometimes very high position is achieved. However, he is not mentally happy.

In Sagittarius: A self made man. Honest with fine manners.

In Capricorn: Vast learning, general family happiness, riches are seen. This is Saturn's own house.

In Aquarius: Learned and philosophical mind. In the early stage mean habits are also present. This is also Saturn's own house.

In Pisces: He is clever and wealthy.

Rahu and Ketu share the qualities of Saturn and Mars, or the qualities with combination.

Note: A planet gets a quality by virtue of its position from Lagna, and by virtue of the Sign also. They are co-related. A bad planet in a bad sign generally gives bad results. A good planet in a bad position and house can only give neutral results. For example, if jupiter happens to be the lord of 5 or 9 if he is in Capricorn can only be neutral. This can be obtained by more experience and in seeing more horoscopes.

9. The Position of Bhavadhipathis in Houses

We have seen the significance of planets in different positions and signs. Now let us examine the results of lords of various places in different bhavas.

In all cases the position of exaltation, Moola Trikona or friendly house or Neecha or evil house has to be noted. The good results may be neutralised if in bad position and the bad results rectified by favourable aspect or combination. Constellation positions also have to be studied.

1st Bhava

1) When lagnadhipathi is in Lagna itself, fortunate life, happiness, wealthy and pushing nature.

2) When in 2nd place, learned, famous, mental peace, noble family traditions, respected.

3) When in 3rd place, happy with brothers, artistic tendencies, authoritative.

4) When in 4th place, wealthy with landed properties, devoted to mother, help from maternal relations.

5) When in 5th place, with good children, religious minded, contact with holy persons, broad minded.

6) When in 6th place sickly, with enemies, debts, worries, cares and anxieties.

7) When in the 7th place, passionate, not realising family responsibilities, travelling, in-laws' property.

8) When in 8th place, subordinate position, suffering from some deformity, unhappy.

9) When in 9th place devoted to father, God fearing, generous, religious minded, noble views, wealthy.

10) When in 10th place, self-made, religious, high position, respected, wealthy. If with favourable combination or aspect also a great leader.

11) When in 11th wealthy, famous, gains etc (11th is 6th to 6th and hence problems, trials, difficulties, unhappiness also).

12) When in 12th place, troubled life, debts, cares anxieties, trials.

2nd Bhava

1) When in lagna, wealthy, famous, long life, generous, sweet talk (this is 12th to 2 and hence, when not well seen difficulties, harshness in speech, defective vision).

2) A strict man of certain principles, fluency of speech, tactful, famous.

3) Unfavourable relationship with brothers, broken education, difficulties.

4) Landed properties, help from maternal relations, business minded, respected by relatives.

5) Well educated, royal life, clever, happy life, sweet speech, bad and unhelpful sons.

6) Always in wants, bad speech, debts. If good aspects are there, there is some relief.

7) Not a favourable life, not happy, submissive to wife and bears all blames. If this is in the lady's horoscope, husband will tease her and married life may not be very pleasant.

8) Harsh speech, troubled life, irresponsible ways, incurring losses.

9) When well aspected property of the father, sweet speech, god fearing nature.

10) Learned, teacher, purohit, Atmagyani, legal advisor, high position, respected.

11) Gain through tactful talk, brokers, wealthy, happy family, above wants.

12) Hard life, debts, enemies and the like.

3rd Bhava

1) This is otherwise 11th from 3rd, good relationship with brothers, artistic views, gains, wealthy condition.

2) Not quite favourable, depending on brothers, not much happy, timid.

3) Devotion to God, authority, high position, happy with brothers, help from them.

4) Happy life, brothers and sisters, good relationship, uncles helpful.

5) Attached to brothers, children religious minded, learned in the Shastras.

6) Quarrel and litigation with brothers, no brothers or sisters, displeasure with brothers.

7) Passionate with Loose character, help from brother's wife or from sisters, dependant.

8) A few or no brothers, litigation, unhappy condition, poor.

9) Devoted to brothers, large family, happy and brave.

10) Dependant upon brothers, unfavourable to brothers, not much pushing.

11) Gains from brothers, happy life.

12) Quarrels, litigations with brothers, loss, unhappy conditions.

4th Bhava

1) Riches, comforts, happy life, devoted to mother, peace of mind.

2) Devoted to mother, maternal property, help from uncles.

3) This is 12th from 4th, ill-health to mother, expenses in family, not quite happy conditions.

4) Lord of kendra in kendrasthana, becomes powerful, happiness, peace of mind, ill health to mother.

5) Helpful sons, comforts, a happy family circle.

6) Unfavourable to mother, no comforts, expenses in family, no peace of mind, family quarrels, no conveyance facility.

7) 4th to 4th is 7th. This is a very strong position, husband or wife from maternal relations, unsteady income, ill health to mother, heavy expenses.

8) Unfavourable to mother, no comforts, misfortune, road accident.

9) Very happy conditions, devotion, orthodox principles, wealthy, lot of cattle.

10) High position, very happy, influential, wealthy condition. If Scorpio is lagna, 4th lord Saturn, 10th position i.e. Leo-Saturn is not favourable there—no peace of mind, very bad for mother, no comforts.

11) Large gains, comforts, bad health of mother, no peace of mind.

12) Poor conditions, no comforts, quarrel or loss through mother, ill health to mother.

5th Bhava

1) Good sons rising to high positions, devotion to God, learned, orthodox, high education when the 5th lord is in lagna. For Cancer the 5th lord is Mars, in Cancer he is Neecha. Mars is held as Yogakarka, however the help from sons is poor unless aspected by Jupiter.

2) In second, high education, sweet speech, earning through literary lines, journalist Putrasthandhipahti in maraka house is not very good for health of children.

3) When in 3rd, sickness to children, broken education, want of discriminating power.

4) While in 4th, when a lord of trikona is in kendra he gets evil powers, breaks in education, not intelligent, expenses.

5) When in 5th much depends upon the planet who happens to be the Lord. Mars, Venus, Saturn, Mercury are evils for Putrasthana. High education, fame, good deeds, respectable positions and the like.

6) When in 6th, sickly children or no children, no benefit from children, poor education, poor conduct.

7) When in 7th, if the lord of 5th in 7th happens to be neecha, wife's health will be affected by delivery, breaks in education, moderate position, not wealthy.

8) When in 8th, sickness to children, poor education, family life very tedious, poor, good deeds of previous births.

9) When in the 9th, very happy life, large family, devoted children, highly religious, very generous, pious, wealthy, charity mind.

10) While in 10th, if Mars as lord of 5th is in 10th, very good position can be expected, happiness, high education to suit the nature of profession, help from children.

11) While in 11th, gains through children, happy home life, contact with superiors, saints or holy persons. 3-6-11 are unfavourable positions also and hence when the lord of 5th by being in 11th happens to be in an evil sign, quite reverse will be the outcome. The putrakaraka Jupiter also decides.

12) While in 12th, danger to mother from delivery, poor education, poverty, unsocial.

6th Bhava

1) When the 6th lord is in lagna, unfavourable conditions in life, some difficulties, enemies, dependant.

2) When in 2nd difficult family life, defective speech, poor eyesight.

3) When in 3rd, quarrel among brothers, debts, disease.

4) When in 4th, unhappy conditions, sickness to mother, poor comforts.

5) When in 5th, unreligious, evil company, poor education, sickness to children.

6) When in 6th, fear of enemies, debts, disease. When an evil planet happens to be the lord of the 6th and when in 6th, exalted life conditions will be very difficult. When the 6th lord in the 6th happens to become Neecha, enemies become powerless, good wealth, moderate health.

7) When in 7th, sickness to wife, later marriage, defective generative organs, poor conduct and characater.

8) When in 8th, from one sickness or the other, debt to the other, theft in house.

9) While in 9th, unfavourable to father, loss of ancestral property, evil doings.

10) While in 10th, gain by illegal ways, punishments, poor conditions.

11) While in 11th, sickness, poverty, litigation, some gains by unfair means.

12) When in 12th, enemies, punishments, fear and the like.

The lord of the 6th has to be in some place and he spoils that Bhava. The evil is rectified when there is a favourable aspect by benefics or when the lord of 6th is Neecha.

7th Bhava

1) When the 7th lord is in Lagna, attracted by fair sex, sinful, passionate dispositions.

2) While in 2nd, helping wife, passionate, submissive.

3) While in the 3rd, bad health to wife or separation,

probability of double marriage, evil connections, poor domestic happiness.

4) When in 4th, adaptable wife, happy family, conveyances and comforts.

5) When in 5th, not good for children, ill health after delivery, artistic views of life, often breaks or hindrances in education.

6) When in 6th, quarrel at house, sickly wife or husband in debts due to family expenses, unhappy conditions.

7) When in 7th, the lord is very powerful and not held very high, if seen in husband's horoscope, family run by wife's income or in-law's help. If seen in wife's horoscope, passionate husband, selfish attitude.

8) When in 8th, unfavourable position, health of the wife will be affected, two marriages, poor income, mounting expenses.

9) When in 9th, happiness, right conduct, devoted to wife or husband, religious minded, early marriage, father's help.

10) When in 10th, early marriage, help from wife side, ill health to wife or husband.

11) When in 11th happiness, property, gain from wife, rich husband, sickness.

12) When in 12th, debts through wife, constant troubles from husband, unhappy married life.

8th Bhava

1) When in lagna, very unfavourable position, accidents, poverty, punishments.

2) When in 2nd, defective speech, harshness in talk, quarrelsome, liar, cheating tendency.

3) When in 3rd, quarrel with brothers or sisters, no brothers, litigation for property.

4) When in 4th, unhappy life, comforts, ill health of mother, road accidents.

5) When in 5th, poor return from children, not attentive in studies, unsteadiness.

6) When in 6th, evil thoughts and actions, accidents, conspiracy, poverty. However when there are good aspects some relief can be seen. 8th house indicates debts, longevity also. Hence, the lord of 8th in 6th is not favourable for long life unless aspected by a benefic like Jupiter. Saturn's positions and Maraka places have to be scrutinized.

7) When in 7th, quarrels in family, debts, ill health.

8) When in 8th, long life, constant troubles, impulsiveness in thought and action.

9) When in 9th, squandering wealth, non-religious, expenses through children, no help from them, very evil thoughts.

10) When in 10th, unsteady profession, subordinate, displeasure with superiors.

11) When in 11th, ill health, displeasure in office, not attentive to work due to poor health, not happy, gain by unfair means.

12) When in 12th, anxiety, cares, losses and the like.

9th Bhava

1) When the 9th lord is in Lagna, high position, generous, religious, learned, respected, devoted to father.

2) When in 2nd house, happiness in family, sweet speech, good education, high family status.

3) When in 3rd house, unfavourable to father and loss in ancestral property, evil doings.

4) When in 4th, devoted to parents, happy family, vehicles, wealthy conditions. A lord of Trikona as kendra position is also not held very high, evil ways, after-thoughts etc.

5) When in 5th, provided it is not neecha place or evil quite favourable, good helping children, respect, famous, wealthy happy family.

6) When in 6th, loss, sickness to children, litigation, unhappy conditions.

7) When in 7th, devoted to wife, happy family, favourable children.

8) When in 8th, loss of property, ill health to father. When Bhagyathipathi is not seen well, a life of poor conditions.

9) When in 9th, happy family, religiousness, good sons, property, generous, large donations to charity institutions.

10) When in 10th, high position, generous, happy family, devoted to father, educated, learned, preacher of religious discourses, purohit, teacher.

11) When in 11th, gains, misunderstandings in family, gain by unfair dealings, losses.

12) When in 12th, very unfavourable situations in life conditions, losses, poor.

10th Bhava

1) When in lagna, magnetic personality, high position, gains, status, large circle of friends.

2) When in 2nd, learned, sweetness and attractive speech, comfort, influential, happy life.

3) When in 3rd, troubles in profession, dependance on brothers, expenses, worried life.

4) When in 4th, this is 7th to 4th, high position, status, respected, vehicles, helping circles or cooperative maternal relation, property.

5) When in 5th high position, enjoyments, fair dealings god fearing, wealthy, learned and cultured.

6) When in 6th, troubles in job, displeasure with superiors, incurring heavy debts, low income, evil gains.

7) When in 7th, ill health to wife, dependant on wife, not held high. The planet of 10th is also to be studied (whether it is Mars or Sun or Venus). Generally very bad for wife or husband. Change of profession (7th is 10th to

10th) is also likely.

8) When in 8th, sickness in family, hindrances in profession, long life, subordinate career.

9) When in 9th, noble views, religiousness, loss of ancestral property, difficult life.

10) When in 10th, ordinary status, influential, helped by persons in authority, charity-minded.

11) When in 11th, gain in profession, wealthy, respected.

12) When in 12th, unsteady profession, poor income, minimum comforts, expenses.

11th Bhava

1) When in Lagna, learned, large gains, wealthy, right conduct, generous.

2) When in 2nd, authoritative, attraction in speech, earning through speech, purohit, preacher, legal advisor.

3) When in 3rd happy, comfortable, brother's help.

4) When in 4th, royal life, high gains, conveyances, happy life, help from maternal side.

5) When in 5th, good helpful children, influential, generous.

6) When in 6th, debts, checks, ill-health, litigation worries.

7) When in 7th, helpful wife or husband, good sons, happiness in family, learned, religious minded.

8) When in 8th, unsteady career, less income, debts, worried life.

9) When in 9th high position, property, devotion to father, help from father, generous minded.

10) When in 10th, respectable profession, gains, comforts, happy life.

11) When in 11th, religious minded, not very wealthy, ordinary status.

12) When in 12th, expenses, less comforts, heavy losses.

12th Bhava

1) When in lagna, laziness, not pushing, spending for comforts.

2) When in 2nd, breaks in education, traveller, disrespected.

3) When in 3rd, loss, misunderstanding with brothers.

4) When in 4th, generous minded, less loss, large family, expenses.

5) When in 5th, loss or expenses through sons, religious, builder of institutions. 12th is Mokshasthana and 5th is Purvapunyasthana.

6) When in 6th, ill health, loss, poor conditions of life.

7) When in 7th, bad company and loss, disease and when 7th lord is well placed, very happy life.

8) When in 8th, litigations, ill health, poverty.

9) When in 9th, litigation, severe loss and debts.

10) When in 10th, troubles in profession, displeasure with superiors, closing of business.

11) When in 11th, gain, noble, long standing activities. Learned. This is opposite to 5th, heavy expenses by children.

12) When in 12th, losses, poor conditions, unhappy life.

It will be seen that Mars, Venus, Mercury, Jupiter and Saturn own more than one house. Hence a bhava lord happens to hold two bhavas. For example, for Aries lagna 2 and 7 are controlled by Venus. When this lord is in 8th or 12th, those two positions are affected, unless this position has beneficial aspects.

A careful study is required. A sign is of 30 degrees. When a planet is in particular place it has to be studied in which degree he is. 9th-28th degree—not much result can be expected. Similarly in a bad bhava when in the last few degrees, no great evil be said. As told earlier, the star position will also reveal their relationship and relative strength.

10. Some Important Points

We have seen how the planets confer good and bad results when in a bhava or sign. Now we shall see some factors regarding Trikona and kendrasthana. This is not complete but certain.

Rule 1: The lords of 5 and 9 do good and the lords of 3-6-11 do evil.

Rule 2: Even when the lords of 5 and 9 are bad by nature they do good and even when bad planets occupy 3-6-11 they do not do good.

Rule 3: In doing good the lord of 9th has more power than 5. In the same way, the lord of 11 does more evil than 6th lord and the 6th lord more than 3rd.

Rule 4: For Aries Lagna Jupiter as lord of 9th can do more benefit than Sun as lord of 5th. So also for Taurus, Jupiter as lord of 11 does more evil.

Rule 5: Good or bad lords of 2 and 12 confer better or worse results in relation to their ownership or kendrasthana.

Rule 6: Lord of 8th is in 12th to Bhagyasthana (9) and hence he is an evil and there is an exception if the lord of 8th happens to be the lord of lagna, he does good. For Aries Mars is also lord of 8th and the Lagnadhipathi. So also for Libra Venus is the Lagnadhipathi and lord of 8th.

Rule 7: As already pointed out 4-7-10 are kendrasthanas. When Jupiter or Venus occupy these positions they get more powers. Next in order are Mercury and Moon.

Mars by virtue of his position as lord of Jivanasthana (10) does not get dosha but does good.

Rule 8: Mars in addition to being the lord of 10th if he is also lord of the 5th, can confer better results.

Rule 9: Jupiter as lord of 4 and 7 for Virgo and Venus as lord of 7 for Aries and Scorpio do bad to the Bhava in which they are. If they are in the same Bhava they do more evil. In the case of Sagittarius, Mercury happens to be the lord of 10 and 7 and he does less evil unless he is badly combined.

Rule 10: Sun and Moon do not get so much evil as Astamadhipathi (8th lord) as in the case of Capricorn or Sagittarius.

Rule 11: Life span is seen from 2, 3, 7, 8 places. Let us see how these places are important. Counted from Lagna 8th place and its 12th place which is 7th are first stage. 8th position to 8th place comes as 3rd house. This is the second stage. 12th position to 3rd 2nd. Thus 2, 3, 7, 8 are factors for life span. Among these 2nd place has more death inflicting power. The lords of 2nd and 7th or the planets in the 2-7- decide more in awarding death than 3-8 places. 2nd house is stronger than the 7th. A planet in 2nd gets more power than its lord. The combining planet in 2 gets more power.

Rule 12: The lords of 3-6-11 are evils. But in certain positions the same lord may become owner of 3 and 10 or 8 and 9 or 10, and 11. In the case of Aquarius Lagna, Mars is lord of 3 and 10 etc.

Please see these charts.

When these lords are combined with favourable planets

12	Lagna 1	II 2	III 3
11			4
10	Rule-II (11)		5
9	8	IV 7	6

Jupiter			
	Examples 6×9	Lagna	

	Mars		
Lagna	Examples 3×10		

	Lagna		
Saturn	Examples 10×11		

			Lagna
Saturn	Examples 8×9		
	Saturn		

or he has aspect of favourable planets, they do not do evil. Merely by virtue of being the lord of Lagna and 8th, a planet does not give only good or bad. For Libra Venus is both lord of Lagna and 8th lord, so also for Aries, Mars. For Cancer Jupiter is lord of 6th and 9th. Is he good as lord of 9th or bad as lord of 6th? When the lord of 6th is in combination with 5th lord there is not much of evil of the 6th lord.

A combination of Mars-Jupiter or Mars-Jupiter-Moon in 1, 5, 9, 10 do good. Hence, in ownership of two houses combination is the deciding factor and also its position.

Take for example Aquarius Lagna. When Mars is in 10th i.e. in Scorpio his strength as lord of 3rd is insignificant. This position of each planet has to be examined carefully.

Rule 12: There are 6 sources of energy for each planet. They are measured in terms of value. They are:

a) Sthana bala or force on account of occupying a particular position as own house or exalted position in a friendly house or Moola Trikona position.

b) Dikbala force by virtue of direction. Jupiter and Mercury get more power in Lagna. Sun and Mars in kendra 10th. Saturn in the 7th and Venus and Moon in 4th.

c) By Motion: Sun is powerful in Uttarayana. Mars, Mercury, Venus, Saturn are powerful in Vakra. Saturn is powerful in vakra or with full moon. Moon is powerful in Capricorn, Aquarius, Pisces, Aries, Taurus and Gemini.

d) Kalabala.

e) Force by aspecting planet

f) Permanent strength.

11. Dasa Periods

Reading the results from Dasa Bhukti is a major factor to decide the course of life for a particular period. Some give predictions for a whole life period and some give only for the current Bhukti and a general sketch for rest of the periods. This depends upon the person's preference and depending upon the same, the Astrologer would undertake the job as desired.

Immediate transfer in job or marriage of son or daughter. Their marriageable age, or building of a house or improvement or relief from sickness etc., can be known by Antara. In Venus Dasa Venus Antara is for a longer duration than in Sun Dasa.

When the Dasa lord is the lord of 5th or 9th Bhava, favourable results are seen. When Saturn or Jupiter Dasas are 4 or 6 respectively, they are unfavourable. The constellation position of the lord of Dasa is also to be studied. Each Dasa has nine sub-divisions or Bhuktis. There seems to be no fixed formula for arriving at conclusions. The results noted in this chapter are furnished in general. Good and bad results are furnished.

Sun Mahadasa - 6 years

1. Sun + sun: (0-3-18 days):

This is not so much a favourable period. Royal displeasure, quarrel in family, ill health, travel, mental uneasiness.

2. Sun + moon: (0-6-0 months):

This is a better period. Promotion in job, expansion of

business, new ventures, respect among relations, and if moon is badly placed, ill health and danger from water.

3. Sun + mars: (0-4-6 days):

Mental tension, ill health, litigation, misunderstanding with relations, loss, worry. When in favourable positions with beneficial aspect, purchase of property, promotions or appointment.

4. Sun + rahu: (0-10-24 days):

When Rahu is in 6, 8, 12 place or combined with evil planet there will be mental worry, loss, failure in undertakings, separation in family, children affected, food poison etc. When in 10 or 11 Royal favour, extra income, freedom from disease.

5. Sun + jupiter: (0-9-18 days):

When jupiter is placed in his own house or Moola Trikona or Trikona or Exalted : Marriage, benefits from friends and relatives, increase of wealth, royal favour, promotion in job, contact with saintly persons, pilgrimage to holy places, victory in court cases. When jupiter is in bad place, in 4 or 7 Neechasthana, the results will be negative and taxing.

6. Sun + saturn: (0-11-12 days):

Sickness to wife and children, loss of money, royal displeasure, transfers in job as punishment, misery, debt.

7. Sun + mercury: (0-10-6 days):

Purchase of ornaments and clothes, favourable trend in education, expansion of business, marriage, pilgrimage. When mercury is in bad position 3, 6, 8, 12 or lord of 4 and 7, mental depression, court troubles, ill health, quarrel, unnecessary travels.

8. Sun + ketu: (0-4-6 days):

This is a period when one must be careful—mental worry, change of residence, family troubles, disease, poison due to insect bitings, headache, misunderstanding among friends. Ketu in 11 with the aspect of jupiter (as lord of 5 or 9) or Venus, advancement in education, name and fame.

9. Sun + venus: (1-0-0 year):

When venus is in Trikona or 2nd benefits from ladies or marriage, Royal favour, promotions, contact with saintly persons, mind towards intense prayers, travel to holy places, purchase of silver or pearls.

Sun is pirtukaraka and hence when in favourable places the period will be moderately good. When in unfavourable, happy results may not come.

Moon Mahadasa - 10 years

1. Moon + moon: (0-10-0 months):

This is a favourable period. Marriage or birth of a child, seeing saints or holy persons, good food, success in undertaking, gain of lost property, change in the living place, good health.

2. Moon + mars: (0-7-0 months):

Normally this is not a favourable period, misunderstanding in the family, loss of wealth, extra expense, ill health due to fire or intsruments, blood troubles.

3. Moon + rahu: (1-6-0 months):

A very taxing period when rahu is combined with lord of 8th, loss of wealth, displeasure with boss, ill health to father or family members, mental agony. When rahu is aspected by benefic, the results are positive in purchasing new house, new vehicle, new venture, political victory.

4. Moon + jupiter: (1-4-0 months):

Generally a favourable period. Promotion in job, meeting holy persons or pilgrimage, child birth, purchase of gold ornaments, marriage etc. When jupiter is in 6, 8, 12 the results will not be so favourable, loss of prestige or position, mental tension.

5. Moon + saturn: (1-7-0 months):

Loss in wealth, mental anxiety, ill health due to bile and misunderstanding with relatives and officer. When saturn is in 3, 6, 11 from Moon, more favourable results can be seen. Either marriage or child birth, new venture in the case of businessmen, new dealings in iron or oil business and gain. Ill health with fatigue will also be the result.

6. Moon + mercury: (1-5-0 months):

Wealth through maternal side, favourable news in dispute, good results in mental activity, Royal favour, happiness through females. If mercury is ill placed, quite contrary results with fear, ill health and mental anxiety.

7. Moon + ketu: (0-7-0 months):

This is an unfavourable period, ill health in family circle, eye troubles, mental worry, displeasure with higher authorities or loss in business. Pilgrimage and blessings of saints likely when ketu is well placed.

8. Moon + venus: (1-8-0 months):

Birth of child or marriage, royal favour, good clothings, sudden wealth, help from in-law's gain in agriculture. When venus is badly placed bad name, evil company, mental worry etc.

9. Moon + sun: (0-6-0 months):

This is a mixed period. Happiness and general prosperity, ill health to parents, general debility, new position or appointment in case of unemployed.

When bright Moon is well placed—gain and happiness, purchase of property etc. and when bad Moon, worry from all sides and loss.

Mars Mahadasa - 7 years

1. Mars + mars: (0-4-27 days):

Misunderstandings between brothers and sisters,

superiors in office, quarrel, loss, ill-health due to excess heat in the body as boils etc.

When Mars is exalted or in own house or in favourable position gain through landed properties or acquisition of house, favourable results in family, litigation, purchase of ornaments and the like.

2. Mars + rahu: (1-0-18 days):

Royal displeasure, mind going towards evil doings, changing the place of living, punishments, loss of cattle, wife, long journey, bad name, fall and injury.

3. Mars + jupiter: (0-11-6 days):

Favourable jupiter indicates pilgrimage, birth of child, promotion, devotion to god. Unfavourable jupiter indicates loss of brothers, loss of money, failure in undertakings, mental worry.

4. Mars + saturn: (1-1-9 days):

Loss of wealth, danger in operation, quarrels, fight, court troubles, displeasure in office and loss of position and mental worry and hard times.

5. Mars + mercury: (0-11-27 days):

Mind diverted towards holy activities, favourable results in education or travel for educational pursuits, marriage, gain in business, respect in society etc. When ill placed, the period will be of mental illness, robbery, money through illegal means, bad name.

6. Mars + ketu: (0-4-27 days):

The period is not a pleasant one. Suffering on account of misunderstandings with brothers or relation or in family, disease due to infection or fire.

7. Mars + venus: (1-2-0 months):

This is a better period when compared to the previous period. Happiness in family, success in matrimonial alliances, religious travels, purchase of property through wife. Victory over enemies. When venus is badly placed, the entire period of Bhukti will give anxiety and mental depression.

8. Mars + sun: (0-4-6 days):
Contact with holy persons or saints, mind occupied with religious thought, long travel, health of the father improving. When sun is badly placed, diseases due to excess heat and mixed events.

9. Mars + moon: (0-7-0 months):
This is a better period. Profit, good health to children, purchase of ornaments, repairs in the living place.

When Mars is the lord of 5 or 9 or 10 or when placed in such position with good benefic aspect the Dasa will give good understanding between brothers and professional betterment and gain.

Rahu Mahadasa - 18 years

1. Rahu + rahu: (2-8-12 days):
Mental anxiety, ill health to wife or other members transfer in the place of working, bad name, poisonous bites, court troubles, leaving home and wandering.

2. Rahu + jupiter: (2-4-24 days):
Promotion in job, child birth or marriage, favourable atmosphere in office, good health, pilgrimage to holy places. Mantra initiation from saints etc. Litigation or court troubles are also likely.

3. Rahu + saturn: (2-10-6 days):
Generally a very unfavourable period, extreme difference of opinion between husband and wife if the 7th bhava is also bad and even divorce or separation, diseases due to pains in joints or excess wind, leaving for remote place.

4. Rahu + mercury: (2-6-18 days):
The previous cloudy period slowly vanishes to enjoy a bright sunshine in life. In the first half of this period

marriage, promotion in the job or expansion of business, new circle of friends etc. In the second part birth of child, obtaining of vehicle, enjoyments in life, evil ways in enjoyments and illegal methods of earning.

5. Rahu + ketu: (1-0-18 days):

This is again a period of strain with disease, ill health due to some poison, wife will become enemy, displeasure with superiors in office, loss of wealth, blame.

6. Rahu + venus: (3-0-0 years):

This will be better period. Purchase of vehicles, wife is source of happiness, marriage or child birth, benefits like promotion, or other favours in the office, gain in agricultural holdings and general happiness. Some trouble from enemies and ill health are also likely.

7. Rahu + sun: (0-10-24 days):

Transfer in job or change in place of working, disease due to excess heat, changing the place of living, educational achievements and charity, mental worry and uneasiness will also prevail.

8. Rahu + moon: (1-6-0 months):

Condition of health changing, some kind of loss through wife, enjoyments in life, travels, foreign travel also likely, financial improvements, gain in lands, death of relatives.

9. Rahu + mars: (1-0-18 days):

This is a period of test indication, displeasure with officers, failure in court cases, loss through brothers or cousins, bad habits, severe mental agony and decrease of mental power.

If Rahu is in 3-6-10 financial improvements are obtained. The aspect of Rahu by a benefic or his combination in a particular bhava decide the nature of result. It is not correct to say that the entire period of 18 years will give trials in life or the man will roll in wealth. When Rahu is in Aries, Taurus, Virgo, Sagittarius, Capricorn gives favourable results. In Gemini, Cancer, Leo, Libra, Scorpio, Aquarius, Pisces gives rather unfavourable results especially in bad bhavas or with evil combination. Sometimes loss of position, imprisonment, abortion, severe loss etc may be the outcome.

Jupiter Mahadasa - 16 years

1. Jupiter + jupiter: (2-1-18 days):

Favourable news in office and promotion, good health, success in activities, pilgrimage, loss of wealth, failures unattachment in family and children.

2. Jupiter + saturn: (2-6-12 days):

Misunderstanding in family and relations, failure in business, debts, litigation, mental uneasiness, funeral ceremonies for others, evil ways and habits, pain in foot or joints.

3. Jupiter + mercury: (2-3-6 days):

Improvement in finance, auspicious ceremonies at home, expansion of business, favour from superiors, mental activities in artistic lines, birth of good child.

4. Jupiter + ketu: (0-11-6 days):

Sacrificing for the sake of others, changing the living place, separation from relations, pilgrimage to holy places, loss in wealth, illness due to poison.

5. Jupiter + venus: (2-8-0 months):

Employment, success or promotion in job or business, happiness at home, improvement in children, purchase of jewels, especially diamond, auspicious ceremonies at home, bad name and difficulties from ladies.

6. Jupiter + sun: (0-9-18 days):

Increase in financial standard, favour from superiors improvement in health, more pious and holy activities.

7. Jupiter + moon: (1-4-0 months):

Children—a source of happiness, marriage or birth of child, purchase or acquisition of property, home comforts, name and fame, benefit in mental activity like writing.

8. Jupiter + mars: (0-11-6 days):

Pilgrimage to holy temples, new ventures and wealth and also loss due to robbery, difficulties in job and displeasure with boss.

9. Jupiter + rahu: (2-4-24 days):

Loss and financial strain, some income from people of low standard, disease, anxiety to wives, mental tension.

Saturn Mahadasa - 19 years

1. Saturn + saturn (3-0-3 days):

Ill health, mental tension, worry from sons, wife and relations. Even servant will not work properly. Some loss is also indicated.

2. Saturn + mercury: (2-8-9 days):

Expansion of education and knowledge, financial improvement, marriage or birth of a child, favourable news in place of work and holy ceremonies at home.

3. Saturn + ketu: (1-1-9 days):

Ill health due to swelling in joints, especially knee joints, loss of money, quarrel with son, fear of poison, trouble through ladies.

4. Saturn + venus: (3-2-0 months):

This is a bright period (when saturn is a yogakaraka and when venus is well placed; this is an excellent period), promotion in job or favourable news at the place of work, happiness in family, success in undertakings, coming of wife's property and victory in disputes.

5. Saturn + sun: (0-11-12 days):

Disease due to poison of blood, theft, affliction in eyes, wife and children badly affected and mental suffering.

6. Saturn + moon: (1-7-0 months):

Loss of property and money, debts, changing of house due to dispute, enemity among relations, death of some important family member.

7. Saturn + mars: (1-1-9 days):

Bad name, wandering or frequent transfers in job, serious illness, loss by theft etc.

8. Saturn + rahu: (2-10-6 days):

Increase of troubles, disease in limb, insect bites, misery in every walk.

9. Saturn + jupiter: (2-6-12 days):

Comparitively this is a better period, purchase of ornaments, physical comforts, success in expected matters, new friends and new position.

Mercury Mahadasa - 17 years

1. Mercury + mercury: (2-4-27 days):

Purchase of home or shifting to more comfortable place, money and help from relatives, learning of astrology or similar subjects. Improvement in conditions of life.

2. Mercury + ketu: (0-11-27 days):

Disease due to excess of bile in the body, unnecessary travels, loss of wealth, mental agony, improvement in education, success in artistic profession can be expected.

3. Mercury + venus: (2-10-0 months):

Religious ceremonies at home, purchase of jewels, marriage or birth of child, family happiness, prosperity to relatives, purchase of landed properties are also liklely. Illegal connections, drinking habit.

4. Mercury + sun: (0-10-6 days):

Royal honour, appointment, vehicles, political career etc. Disease in stomach, fire accidents, sickness to wife, acquisition of some wealth.

5. Mercury + moon: (1-5-0 months):

Health troubles, disputes through ladies, gain through women, jewels, general ill will of relations.

6. Mercury + mars: (0-11-27 days):

Some benefits from superiors, disease due to insect bite, neighbours becoming enemies, visiting house of ill fame, punishments by superiors, mental anxiety.

7. Mercury + rahu: (2-6-18 days):

Evil and bad connections with ladies, change in position, failure in cases, money from friends, disease due to indigestion and the like, acquisition of divine knowledge.

8. Mercury + jupiter: (2-3-6 days):

Some benefits from superiors, birth of son, closeness of relations, wife becoming more attached, ill feeling with relations, quarrel, ill health, loss of wealth, misunderstanding with father or son and the like.

9. Mercury + saturn: (2-8-9 days):

Diseases, debts, scandal, money from illegal sources, failure in land holdings or failure in iron or oil business. Good actions like building temples or charities or pilgrimage.

Ketu Mahadasa - 7 years

1. Ketu + ketu: (0-4-27 days):

Mental worry due to son or wife, loss of money, poison fear, a general setback and check in life.

2. Ketu + venus: (1-2-0 months):

Success in any undertaking, birth of child, ill health to children, fever or dysentery.

3. Ketu + sun: (0-4-6 days):

Check in business, expansion of knowledge, uneasiness, travel, health of wife giving anxiety and worry.

4. Ketu + moon: (0-7-0 months):

Financial improvements, loss, mental uneasiness, disease through water or cold, troubles form children.

5. Ketu + mars: (0-4-27 days):

A general anxiety about children, quarrels in family, increase of enemies, punishments, death, operation in the body.

6. Ketu + rahu: (1-0-18 days):

Royal punishments, blood poison, loss of wealth or property, loss in business, visiting prostitute for pleasure.

7. Ketu + jupiter: (0-11-6 days):

Contact with persons of high status, happiness through wife, marriage, increase in holdings, profits in business.

8. Ketu + saturn: (1-1-9 days):

Prison-like conditions, loss of money in many ways, strained feelings with relations, exile to far off places, change of house.

9. Ketu + mercury: (0-11-27 days):

Money from mental pursuits, children giving worry and anxiety, failure of ideas or plans, fear from relations etc.

When Ketu is well placed or aspected by jupiter or Venus holding Trikona position—gives pilgrimage to holy places, dip in sacred rivers, finishing of *prarthana* in family etc. Better results are gained when ketu is in Gemini, Leo, Libra, Sagittarius or Pisces. A trip to Varanasi or Remeswaram during ketu dasa is highly beneficial. The mind will get better concentration.

Venus Mahadasa - 20 years

1. Venus + venus: (3-4-0 months):

This is the longest period in life when placed in signs other than Cancer, Leo, Virgo, Scorpio, Venus does give better results. A general easiness will prevail in life conditions, increase in finances, fame, birth of male child.

2. Venus + sun: (1-0-0 year):

This is not so much a favourable period. General anxiety, troubles in family, quarrel, damage to property and wealth.

3. Venus + moon: (1-8-0 months):

Gain through ladies, expansion of mental activity, vehicles, success in undertakings, intense devotion to God, nervous troubles due to excess sexual pleasure and trouble through ladies.

4. Venus + mars: (1-2-0 months):

Increase of family holdings, marriage, wealth through ladies, materialistic outlook, disease of eye or bile.

5. Venus + rahu: (3-0-0 years):

Change of place of living, getting property by lottery or race or by unexpected ways, silent prayers, name and fame.

6. Venus + jupiter: (2-8-0 months):

Help from persons in rank, patronage from wife and children. Royal honour and wealth. When jupiter is in 6, 8, 12 or a maraka—unnecessary travels, failure, general disgust in life.

7. Venus + saturn: (3-2-0 months):

Disease due to evil habits, bad company, loss of health and money.

8. Venus + mercury: (2-10-0 months):

Marriage, success in litigation, increase in financial standard, children giving mental satisfaction, ailments in the body.

9. Venus + ketu: (1-2-0 months):

Pilgrimage, worship, visiting saints, good education to children, danger from animals, weakness of body, anxiety but the end will be in happiness.

Note: When a person lives 120 years all the dasas will operate. Normally due to present day living conditions, one gets tired by the age of 60 or 65. Hence, only certain dasas are operative, some may not have saturn dasa at all.

A person born on Revathi with mercury beginning will be over 60 when Mars is operative. When the beginning dasa is jupiter, most probably by the end of Venus Dasa he will be 79 and even Sun dasa is not likely.

When the beginning dasa is Rahu with balance of major time in birth, say 15 years, the life will reflect on Rahu, Jupiter, Saturn, unless jupiter is well placed and perfect yogakaraka life will be one of continuous trivials only since Rahu 15, Jupiter 16, Saturn 19 which add to 50 years.

Persons having major period in Mercury as beginning dasa, say 15 years, Ketu-7, Venus-20, Sun-6, Moon-10, Mars-7 are 65 or so. Neither Rahu nor Saturn is operative in this case.

God's creation is so well balanced that Dasa or Bhukti are so intermingled that at no time a man is absolutely free.

If the Dasa and Bhukti periods are studied, it will be seen the periods are equal. For example, in Sun dasa venus bhukti is one year. In venus Dasa sun bhukti is also one year. In Jupiter dasa Rahu bhukti is 2-4-24 days. Similarly in Rahu dasa Jupiter Bhukti is 2-4-24.

It is generally believed that no Dasanathan (Dasa's starting period) can confer either good or bad but continue the events of the previous period only i.e. status-quo.

For example, if Saturn dasa has done very bad results and the next mercury dasa in his bhukti does not at all make sudden changes in everything. Every planet gives the results in accordance with the combination or aspects. If jupiter has mars combination during Jupiter Dasa-Mars bhukti will also do good. If Moon has the beneficial aspect of Mars during Moon Dasa Mars bhukti, favourable trend will prevail. The good results during the Dasa of a Trikonasthana planet will be given in the Bhukti of the other Trikona lord. Similarly when Dasanathan is an evil even when the Bhukthinathan is a favourable planet, cannot do good.

There is a golden saying in astrology: "Astrology can give only a hint but it cannot exactly say what can happen, except the creator Brahma, who else can know."

12. Yogas

Human life falls under two grand divisions. Yogas and Avisthas, or fortunes and misfortunes. Yogas include success in every line and Avisthas or misfortunes inlcude all sorts of sorrows etc. A yoga is formed by more than one planet. The nature of a planet is of three types viz. benefics, malefic and neutral.

According to the natural classification benefics are Jupiter, Venus, well associated Mercury and waxing Moon and malefics are the Sun, Mars, Saturn, evil-associated Mercury and waning Moon. The benefics or benefic lords are (1) lord of Lagna, (2) lords of 5th and 9th, and (3) lords of kendras or quadrants when they are natural malefics. The malefics are (1) the lords of the 3rd, 6th and 11th and (2) lords of kendras when they are natural benefics. The lords of the 2nd and 12th may be termed neutral because they give good and bad results according to their other conjunctions. The 8th lord is a malefic according to Jataka Chandrika but for all practical purposes, he may be taken as a neutral. The above can be classified thus:

Benefics: Lord of 1, lords of 5 and 9, and lords of 4, 7, 10 if they are natural malefics.

Malefics: Lords of 3, 6 and 11. Lords of 4, 7, and 10 if they are natural benefics.

Neutrals: Lords of 2, 8 and 12.

Of course, the 8th lord is supposed to be evil unless he be the Sun or the Moon. We shall avoid controversies and assume that the 8th lord is neutral for the purpose of interpreting yogas.

In the above list of benefics, malefics and neutrals, we have completely forgotten to take into account the influence due to a double lordship. Thus for Aquarius, Mars owns the 10th a quadrant is good. In addition to the 10th he owns the 3rd also which is bad. In other words, Mars, a natural malefic becomes a benefic lord by virtue of owning a kendra. Mars is 'influenced' by his own ownership of the 3rd house. It will be seen that excepting Sun and Moon all other planets own two houses each so that whether a planet is a benefic or malefic, can be judged only when both the lordships are taken into account. The nature of a lord is influenced by two factors viz: (1) the other lordship and (2) association. The other lordship varies with regard to different ascendants. When pisces is Lagna, Mars owns 2nd and 9th houses while he owns 1st and 8th when Aries is Lagna. Thus the 'Ascendant' is of the utmost importance while deciding the benefics and malefic lords. Before attempting to interpret yogas properly the strength of the various planets have to be noted. A yoga is formed by atleast two planets. Though there are three hundred important combinations, the author wishes to name a few commonly understood yogas which are given below:

1. **Gajakesari yoga:** If Jupiter is in a kendra from the Moon, the combination goes under the name Gajakesari. This indicates many relations polite and generous, builder of villages and towns or magistrate over them; will have a lasting reputation even long after death.

2. **Sunapha yoga:** If there are planets (excepting the Sun) in the second house from moon, Sunapha is caused. This indicates self-earned property, king, ruler or his equal, intelligent, wealthy and good reputation.

3. **Anapha yoga:** If there are planets in the 12th from moon, Anapha yoga is formed. This indicates, well formed organs, majestic appearance, good reputation, polite, generous, self-respect, fond of dress and sense pleasures. In later life, renunciation and austerity.

4. **Dhuradhara yoga:** If there are planets on either side of the moon, the combination goes under the name

of Dhuradhara. This indicates the native is bountiful. He will be blessed with wealth and conveyances.

5. **Kemadruma yoga:** When there are no planets on both sides of the Moon kemadruma yoga is formed. This indicates the person will be dirty, sorrowful, doing unrighteous deeds, poor, dependant, a rogue and a swindler.

6. **Chandra Mangala yoga:** If Mars cojoins the Moon, this yoga is formed. This indicates earnings through unscrupulous means, a seller of women treating mother harshly and doing mischief to her and other relatives.

7. **Adi yoga:** If benefics are situated in the 6th, 7th and 8th from the Moon, their yoga is formed. This indicates, the person will be polite and trustworthy, will have an enjoyable and happy life, surrounded by luxuries and affluence, will inflict defeat on his enemies, will be healthy and live a long life.

8. **Chatussagara yoga:** Is caused when all the kendras are occupied by planets. This indicates, the person will earn good reputation, be equal to a ruler, have a long and prosperous life, be blessed with good children, health and his name will travel far and wide.

9. **Vasumathi yoga:** If benefics occupy the upachayas (3, 6, 10 and 11) either from the ascendant or from the Moon, this goes under Vasumathi yoga. This indicates the person will not be a dependant but will always command plenty of wealth.

10. **Rajalakshana yoga:** Jupiter, Venus, Mercury and the Moon should be in lagna or they should be placed in kendra. This indicates the native will possess an attractive appearance and he will be endowed with all the good qualities of high personage.

11. **Vanchana Chora Bheethi yoga:** The lagna is occupied by a malefic with Gulika in trines: or Gulika is associated with the lords of the kendras and Trikonas: or the lords of Lagna is combined with Rahu, Saturn or ketu. This

indicates the Native will always entertain feelings of suspicion towards others around him. He is afraid of being cheated, swindled and robbed. Here, three sets of combinations can be noted. They are—

(a) The ascendant must have an evil planet with Gulika disposed in the 5th or 9th.

(b) Gulika should be associated with the lords of 1, 4, 7, 10, 5 and 9.

(c) Lord of lagna should join Rahu or Saturn or Ketu.

In all these cases, the person will not only have fears from cheats, rogues and theives but he will also have huge material losses.

12. **Sakata yoga:** The Moon in the 12th, 6th or 8th from Jupiter gives rise to Sakata Yoga. This indicates the native loses fortune and may regain it. He will be ordinary and insignificant. He will suffer from poverty, privation and misery. He will be stubborn and hated by relatives.

13. **Amala yoga:** The 10th from the moon or Lagna should be occupied by a benefic planet. This indicates the person will achieve lasting fame and reputation. His character will be spotless and he will lead a prosperous life.

14. **Parvata yoga:** Benefics being disposed in kendras, the 6th and 8th houses should either be unoccupied or occupied by benefic planets. This indicates the person will become wealthy, prosperous, liberal, charitable, humorous and head of a town or village. He will be passionate. According to some, Parvata is also caused if the lords of lagna and the 12th are in mutual kendras.

15. **Kahala yoga:** Lords of the 4th and the 9th houses should be in kendras from each other and the lord of Lagna should be strongly disposed. This indicates the native will be stubborn, not well informed, daring, head of a small army and a few villages.

16. **Vesi yoga:** If planets other than the Moon occupy the 2nd from the Sun, vesi yoga is formed. This indicates

the person will be fortunate, happy, virtuous, famous and aristocratic. If malefics occupy the 2nd from the Sun, papavesi is caused while subhavesi is given rise to by the presence of benefic planets.

17. **Vasi yoga:** Planets other than the Moon occupying the 12th from the Sun gives rise to Vasi yoga. This indicates the subject will be happy, prosperous, liberal and favourite of the ruling classes. Here also papa and subha vasi yogas are also formed.

18. **Obhayachari yoga:** If planets other than the Moon are present on either side of the Sun, Obhayachari is caused. This indicates the person will be an eloquent speaker. He will have well proportioned lilmbs, will take delight in everything, will be liked by all; wealthy and famous.

19. **Panchamahapurusha yogas:**

    a. **Hamsa yoga:** Jupiter should occupy a kendra which should be his own house or exalted sign. This indicates his legs will have the markings of conch, lotus, fish and ankusa. He will possess handsome body, he will be liked by others, he will be righteous in disposition and pure in mind.

    b. **Malavya yoga**: Venus should occupy a quadrant which should be his own house or exaltation sign. This indicates the person will have a well developed physique, will be strong minded, wealthy, happy with children and wife, will possess vehicles endowed with clean sense organs and renowned and learned.

    c. **Sasa yoga:** If Saturn occupies a kendra which should be his own house or exaltation sign. This indicates the native will have many servants. His character will be questionable. He will be head of a village or town or even a king, will covet others' riches and will be wicked in disposition.

    d. **Ruchaka yoga:** Mars should be exalted in a kendra or occupy a kendra which should be his own house. This indicates the native will have good physique, famous, well-versed in ancient lore, king or an equal to a King conforming to the traditions and customs. He will have a ruddy complexion, attractive body, charitable disposition, wealthy, long lived and leader of an army.

    e. **Bhadra yoga:** The disposition of Mercury in a kendra which should be identical with his own or exaltation sign. This indicates the person will have a lion-like face, well developed chest, well proportioned limbs, will be taciturn, will help relatives and will live upto a good old age.

20. **Budha-Aditya yoga:** If Mercury combines with the Sun the combination goes under the name of the Budha-Aditya yoga. This indicates highly intelligent, skilful in all works, good reputation, personal respect and surrounded by all comforts and happiness.

21. **Mahabhagya yoga:** In the case of a man, when the birth is during day time the Sun, the Moon and the Lagna should be in odd signs. In the case of women, when the birth is during night, the Sun, the Moon and the Lagna must be in even signs. This indicates a male born under this yoga will have good character, will be a source of pleasure to others, will be liberal, generous, famous, a ruler or an equal to him and lives to a good old age. A female born in this combination will be blessed with long lived children and wealth and will be of a good conduct.

22. **Pushkala yoga:** The lord of the sign occupied by the Moon (who should be associated with lord of Lagna) should be in a kendra or in the house of an intimate friend aspecting Lagna and at the same time, Lagna should be occupied by a powerful planet. This indicates wealth, sweet speech, famous, honoured by the king and a lord.

23. **Lakshmi yoga:** If the lord of Lagna is powerful and the lord of the 9th occupies own or exaltation sign identical with a kendra or Trikona, Lakshmi yoga is caused. This indicates the person will be wealthy,

noble, learned, a man of high integrity and reputation, handsome appearance, a good ruler, and enjoying all the pleasures and comforts of life.

24. **Guru-chandala yoga:** Conjunction of Jupiter with Rahu causes this yoga. Such persons suffer poverty. They do not have peace of mind. The yoga caused by ketu and jupiter helps those who are inclined to practise yoga. They develop suspicious nature and not likely to trust others. The effects are severe in case of females.

25. **Kalasarpa yoga:** Rahu and ketu, the shadowy planets are responsible for creating kalasarpa yoga. It has the following essential conditions to form:

    1. Rahu must be in one of the six signs and Ketu should be in one of the last six houses.
    2. The other seven planets be hemmed between Rahu and Ketu.
    3. There must not be conjunction either with Rahu or Ketu.

Rahu is head and Ketu is tail—both always retrograde. So when the seven planets are between head and tail, this yoga is formed.

It is experienced that many talented persons who were intelligent and capable are born under this yoga. But they have a chequered career, rise to highest order, suffer miseries and even death due to this yoga. Pt. Jawahar Lal Nehru had this yoga in his birth chart. The horoscope of Pakistan has this yoga also.

Some scholars are of the view that if all the seven planets are between Ketu and Rahu this yoga does not form.

The effect of this yoga is that the native gets success in his life after great struggle but there is downfall which gives considerable setbacks, failures and miseries etc. This yoga gives effects generally in major and minor periods of Rahu and Ketu. In the individual birth chart when this yoga is present, shows disturbed and unsuccessful married life, chequered career and obstacles in business, unhealthy relations with every type of partner. This is supposed to make the native suffer till one third of his life i.e. upto 35 to 40 years.

When this yoga is formed in the country's birth chart, Lagna to the 7th house indicates disharmony, strained relations between ruler and public.

The kalasarpa yoga exists and is not cancelled, even though if one or two planets join Rahu or Ketu. The native has to experience the effects of such yoga. Five successive houses behind the nodes should be vacant.

In some cases we have found that when this yoga exists the Ascendant falls outside the axis of nodes. So it does not matter whether the ascendant falls outside or inside the axis of the nodes.

When some planets conjunct Rahu or Ketu beyond ORB, the malefic effects decrease but not spared completely. Malefic effects of Saturn and Mars dominate while benefic aspects of Jupiter and other benefic planets are not feasible. That is why it is malefic.

13. Issue

Birth of worthy children is the legitimate object of marriage which makes an individual's personality complete. Our Dharma Sastras lay down that to propagate the lineage is one of the duties of man, as otherwise he would become a debtor to his ancestors. Hence, the consummation of wedlock is realised in the birth of a son. One must therefore be very fortunate to have good and long lived children. All the details of children are read as you know from the 5th Bhava mainly and the 9th Bhava as well as from their lords and the planets connected with them. In this one who is the karaka or significator of issue also must be well placed and strong. In this connection you will do well to remember the sign of the zodiac that is termed 'Alpasutha' or 'few children'. They are Taurus, Leo, Virgo and Scorpio.

A person can expect good children under the following conditions:

1. Jupiter and the lords of 5th house counted from ascendant and the Moon should be well placed.
2. The 5th house/bhava itself be co-joined with or aspected by benefics or lords of auspicious houses (i.e. other than the 6th, 8th and 12th).
3. The lords of the Ascendant and the 5th house should be cojoined in mutual reception (i.e. exchange houses) or aspect each other.
4. Both Jupiter and the lord of the 5th house in Vaisesikamsa and are aspected by the lord of the 9th house. One is blessed with a son early in life, if the lords of Vth be in a kendra or kona and cojoined with benefics.

Similarly, examine the 5th bhava counted from Jupiter as well. If there are malefics in the house as well as in the two mentioned above (i.e. 5th house from the Ascendant and the Moon) or if malefics aspect or surround them and if the lords of these 5th houses are posited in inauspicious houses, without benefic aspect or association, one cannot be blessed with issue. Now let us suppose that the lord of the 5th house who is a natural malefic occupies it. Would it destroy the house? No, because the owner of a house cannot and will not destroy it. So, birth of children is assured in that case. On the other hand, the presence of a malefic in 5th house owned by a benefic will harm progeny.

1. If one of the signs designated as Alpasutha happens to be the 5th house, one will have no issue or have it very late in life.
2. If the Sun be in such a sign happening to be the 5th house, Saturn in the 8th and Mars in the Lagna, one might expect to have a child with difficulty in life.

Now you must be anxious to know the rules for predicting birth of sons and daughters. The following govern the male births:

The 5th bhava and/or its lord (who being a male planet himself) should be situated in a male Sign or Amsa and/or be in conjunction with or aspected by male planets.

For a female birth substitute the word 'female' for 'male' in rule 1 above.

Conception is likely to take place when Sun, Venus for men, and Mars and the Moon for women are possessed of strength and pass through Apacaya houses (i.e. other than the 3rd, 6th, 10th and 11th houses) identical with their own Signs or Amsa.

The following planetary combinations indicate the loss of children and issuelessness:-

1. The lords of the Vth house should be in depression, in inimical house or be eclipsed, or be in conjunction with the lords of the 6th, 8th and 12th houses without any benefic aspect or conjunction.
2. Mars and Saturn should aspect the 5th house (No issue).

3. The lords of the 7th house should be in the 5th house (No wife, no issue).

The following planetary combination lead to the extinction of the family:

1. Malefics occupying the 6th, 8th and 12th houses counted from the house of issue.
2. The 4, 7 and 10th houses being owned respectively by a malefic, Venus and the Moon.
3. The Lagna, 5th, 8th and 12th houses tenented by malefics.

Adoptions

The following planetary combinations indicate a son by adoption:

1. The 5th Bhava owned by Saturn or Mercury being aspected by or cojoined with Mandi or Saturn.
2. The lord of Vth house being weak and having connection whatsoever with the lords of the 1st and 7th houses.

14. Matrimony

Male and female are but the two aspects, or two sides of Nature. Hence, it is natural for them to be united. Human marriage is but a gross reflection of those grand spiritual union. The ancients have called therefore, the wife, a housewife, a minister, a friend, a slave etc. She is also the goddess of the house, encouraging her husband to earn wealth, name and fame. She stands by him in times of crisis. Though marriages are made in heaven, human beings are not aware of the would-be partners in life. Hence, they search for a suitable person to fill the vacancy. Their anxiety is all the greater as the selection is made but once in a life time.

The wife will be long lived and good if the lord of the VIIth house counted from the Ascendant or the Moon be well placed, well associated and well aspected. So is the case when this Bhava itself occupies or aspected by the lord of the 9th house, benefics or its own lord. The significator of this Bhava viz, Venus, too should be strong, in a good house receiving benefic aspects. On the other hand, if the Bhava and its lord are afflicted i.e. by the occupation of and aspect, the result would not be happy. There will be misery in conjugal life or loss of wife in case there are malefics in the 12th, 4th and 8th from Venus, or if Venus is cojoined with, aspected or surrounded by malefics. The following planetary combinations (yogas) lead to undesirable effects with regard to conjugal life.

1. The lord of the 7th Bhava be in 5th house—loss of wife or progeny.
2. Lord of 5th or 8th house is in 7th—same as above.
3. Weak Moon in 5th and malefics in 1st, 7th and 12th houses—wifeless and childless.

4. The Sun and Rahu in 7th—loss of wealth as a result of association with women.
5. Venus in Scorpio which is 7th house—loss of wife.
6. Mercury in Taurus identical with 7th—same as above.
7. Jupiter in the 7th in depression—as above.

The following yogas lead to good results—

1. The lord of the 8th house be in a kendra, owned by a benefic aspected by a benefic or occupying a benefic Amsa—the wife will be chaste and dutiful and coming from a noble family.
2. Cancer be the 7th house occupied by Mars and Saturn—the wife would be beautiful and chaste.
3. The lord of this Bhava be cojoined with the lord of the Ascendant—the wife would be excellent.
4. The lord of the Ascendant be in the 7th house along with a benefic—the wife belongs to a good family.
5. The Moon occupying the 1st or 7th house in her own or exaltation sign and aspected by a benefic—wife is virtuous.
6. The 7th house falling in a benefic sign or Amsa (still better if aspected by benefics)—wife is virtuous.
7. The 7th house, its lord and venus be all in even signs and be bright, and strong—the wife will be very good.
8. The lords of 2, 7 and 12 houses occupying kendras or konas and being aspected by Jupiter, or benefics occupying the 2nd, 7th and 11th houses counted from the lord of the 7th house—the subject will give all happiness to the wife.

Compatability of horoscopes

People generally say that a person who is Mangali or has Kuja dosha cannot be matched with a girl who does not possess this Dosha. Person who has this trouble will adversely affect the life of the partner. Hence, they look for girls with Kuja Dosha for counteracting the same in the boy's chart. It is to be remembered that the Girl should not have this trouble more than the boy. The reason is quite obvious. While matching the horoscopes, care should be taken to ascertain the longevity, Dasas, relationship of the Dasa lords, ending periods of the dasas etc. in the two charts. Before proceeding further let us know what Kuja dosha is. If Mars is posted in the 12th, 2nd, 4th, 7th and 8th houses form the Lagna, Kuja dosha is brought into existence. The above places are also to be counted from the Moon and as well as from Venus. But in my opinion counting should be from Lagna only. If the boy alone has this he will lose his wife soon. Likewise see if there are malefics in the 2nd and the 7th houses. For, they too are harmful to the wife. It is also bad for the wife if Mars occupies the 7th house and the amsa belonging to venus. The native will be passionately attached to his wife, if the lord of the 7th house is aspected or cojoined with venus, or occupies a house owned by venus, the same effect has to be predicted, if the lord of the 2nd house too is under similar circumstances; or if the lord of the 10th house occupies the 7th along with the venus.

When major points of agreement is there the married life will be moderately well off. Normally, a married life has to extend for atleast 40 years and with atleast one male child, though the birth of a male child is God's gift.

Sashtiabadpurthi—60th birthday of husband is an important function for the couples. The wish of any old lady is that she should die before her husband, as 'sumangali'. No lady wishes for widowhood. Hence, certain agreements are necessary.

There are ten such agreements factors in vogue. They are as follows:

1. Star order number of boy and girl 2. Gana 3. Mahendra 4. Stree Dirgha 5. Yoni 6. Rasi 7. Lord of Rasi 8. Vasya 9. Rajju and 10. Vedha. However, additional one Nadi is also included.

After getting all these verified finally there is percentage of agreement charts and the percentage is verified from them. A minimum of 18 points say 50% is supposed to be good for agreement. Hence, the readers are requested to refer to the book, written by the author of *'Marriage matching—Astrologically'* published by the same publishers which gives a detailed information on the marriage matching and compatability, and other related aspects.

It is not enough to see these agreements factors alone. The horoscopic position of planets should also be scrutinised. Importance to 4, 5, 7, 8, 9 bhavas are essential. When there is a defect in one horoscope and it is rectified in the other then there will be some smooth running since the adverse in one will be rectified by the other. Some examples and case-studies are given for information and easy understanding.

Examples

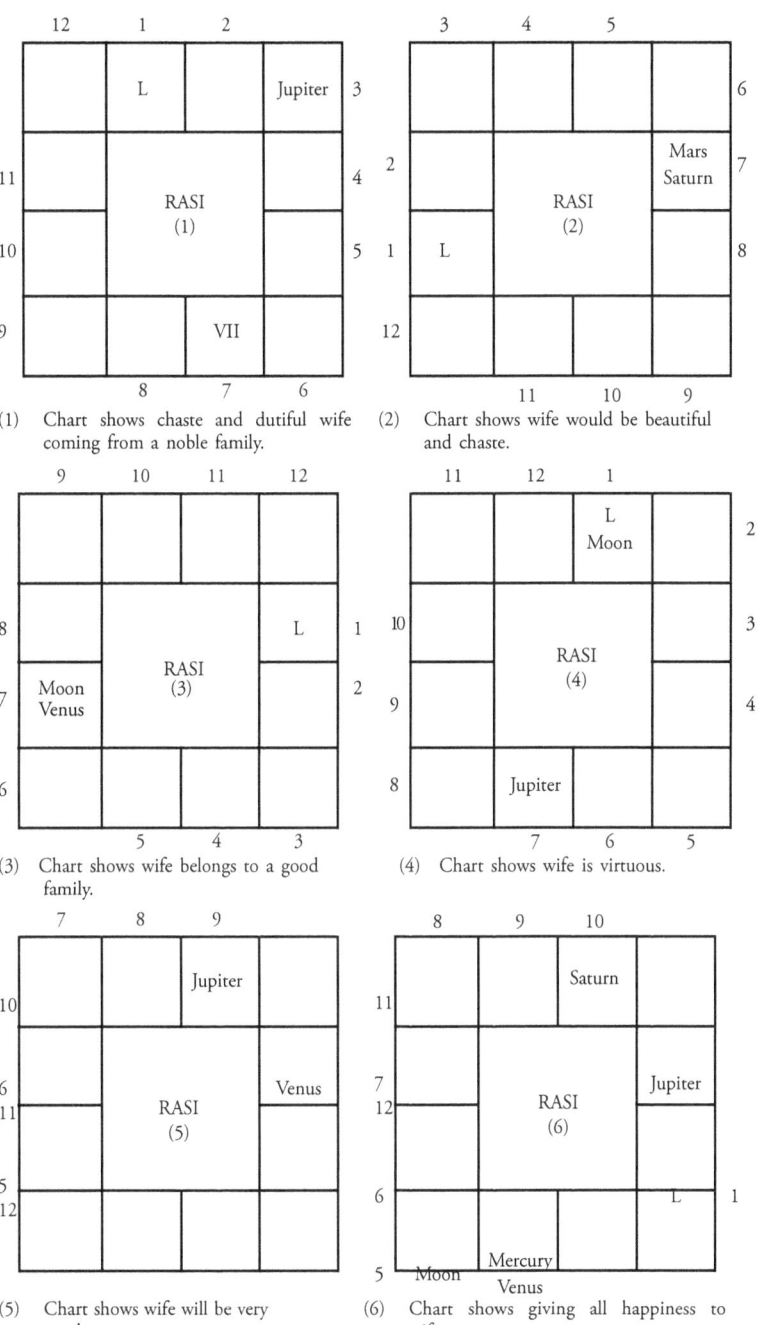

(1) Chart shows chaste and dutiful wife coming from a noble family.

(2) Chart shows wife would be beautiful and chaste.

(3) Chart shows wife belongs to a good family.

(4) Chart shows wife is virtuous.

(5) Chart shows wife will be very good.

(6) Chart shows giving all happiness to wife.

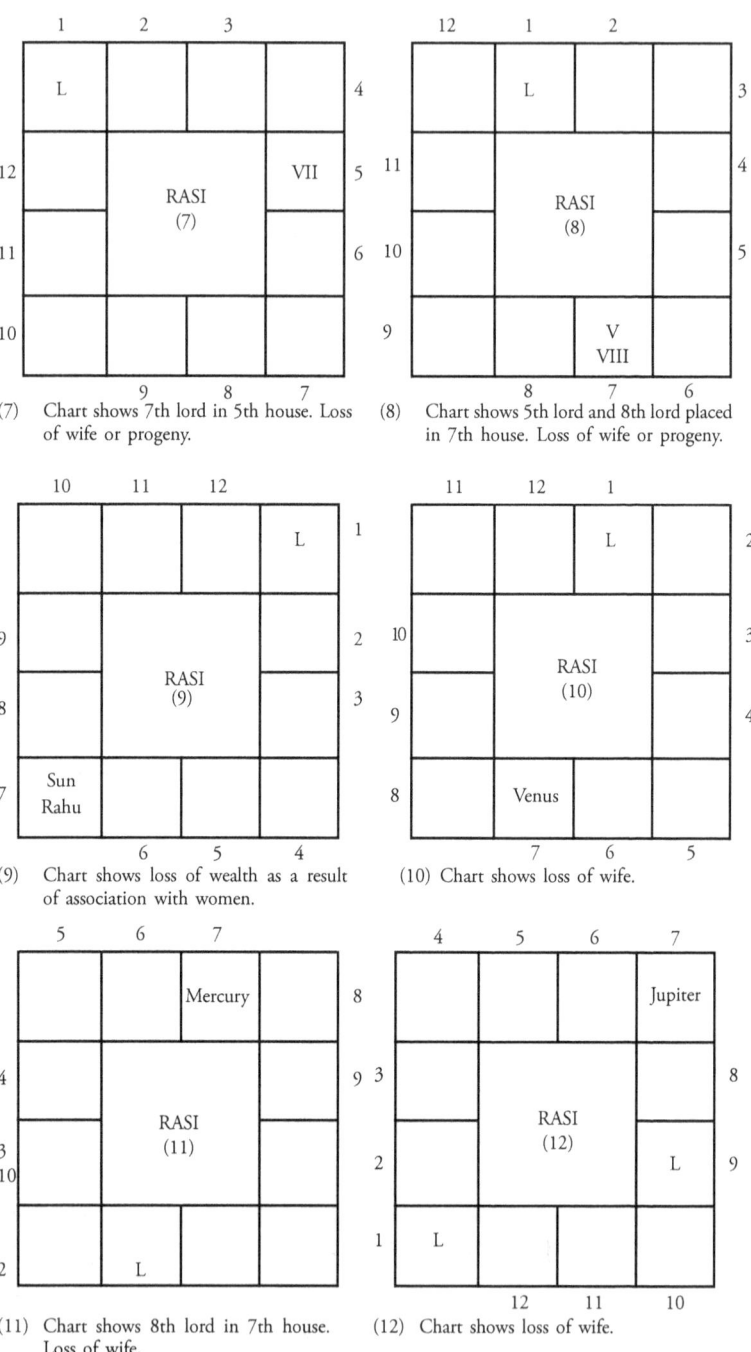

(7) Chart shows 7th lord in 5th house. Loss of wife or progeny.

(8) Chart shows 5th lord and 8th lord placed in 7th house. Loss of wife or progeny.

(9) Chart shows loss of wealth as a result of association with women.

(10) Chart shows loss of wife.

(11) Chart shows 8th lord in 7th house. Loss of wife.

(12) Chart shows loss of wife.

Case-1

11	12	1		
	L	Ketu	2	
10	RASI	Jupiter	3	
9 Moon			4	
8 Mars Rahu	Venus	Mercury Saturn	Sun	
	7	6	5	

Mercury Saturn Ketu			
	Navamsa		Sun Moon Venus
			L Jupiter
Mars			Rahu

The presence of the 7th lord in the 8th and Saturn's aspect on it together with Rahu's association indicates loss of husband as 'Vaidhavya' during Mars, Rahu Dasa. The native married in August 1976. Her husband died in a drowning accident in June 1977, Just 10 months after marriage. Both events occurred in Venus Bhukti or Rahu Dasa. Rahu is in the 8th house afflicting the 8th house with Mars and Saturn. There is a classical dictum that 'If Rahu combines with Mars and Saturn occupies the 7th or the 8th house early widowhood

Case-2

7	8	9		
Sun Saturn	Venus Moon	Ketu		10
6 Mercury	RASI			11
5 Jupiter				12
4	Rahu Mars		L	
	3	2	1	

L Rahu		Mercury	
	Navamsa		Venus
Jupiter			Sun Saturn
	Moon		Mars Ketu

Although the 7th lord Jupiter is strongly placed, his exchange of house with the 5th lord Saturn is not desirable as it can deny marriage or progeny. Further the affliction of the 8th house from the moon is heavy resulting in a Vaidhavya yoga.

Case-3

	3	4	5	6
		Ketu	Jupiter	
2	Moon	RASI	7	
1	L		8	Saturn
12		Mars Rahu	Sun Mercury	Venus
	11	10	9	

	Jupiter Saturn	
Rahu	Navamsa	Venus
Moon		Ketu
Mars	Sun Mercury	L

The 7th house both from lagna and the Moon being free of malefic influences gives a happy married life.

Case-4

	7	8	9	
	Mars		Jupiter Saturn	
6	Ketu	RASI		Moon	11
5	Venus		Rahu	12
4		Sun Mercury		L
	3	2	1	

L	Venus	Ketu	
Mars Sun		Navamsa	
Saturn			Jupiter
	Rahu Mercury		Moon

The 7th lord in the 9th house gives a well placed partner. Saturn's association as the 5th and 6th lords gives the partner a rigid and conservative nature while the position of Mars as a malefic lord causes tensions and quarrels in married life due to temperamental differences.

Case-5

4	5	6	7				
	Ketu			Rahu Sun		Venus Mercury	Moon
3 Moon	RASI		8	Mars	Navamsa		
2			9	Saturn			L Jupiter
1 L Venus	Saturn	Sun Mercury Rahu	Mars Jupiter				Ketu
	12	11	10				

Both from Lagna and Chandra Lagna 7th lord is afflicted by Rahu. Further from the lagna 7th lord is in 11th with Rahu. This results in a husband who was already married at the time of marriage with another.

Case-6

	2	3	4					
	Rahu		Moon Saturn		5		Saturn	Venus	
1	L	RASI	Sun	6	Sun Rahu	Navamsa		
12			Mars Mercury Venus	7				Mercury Moon Ketu
11		Jupiter	Ketu		L	Jupiter	Mars	
	10	9	8					

The native is happily married to a devoted and chaste wife with religious outlook. Kaltrakaraka venus is in the 7th house with two other planets. A stable marriage. This is because Venus although in kendra in the 7th, is not good, hence in this case the stigma is countered as venus is yogakaraka.

Case-7

		Jupiter	
	RASI		Ketu
Rahu			Moon
Sun Venus Mercury		Mars Saturn	L

Houses (Rasi): 7, 8, 9, 10, 11, 12, 1, 2, 3, 4, 5, 6

	Mercury	Venus	
L Saturn			Ketu Sun
Rahu Mars	Navamsa		
Moon			Jupiter

The strength of the 7th lord and kalatrakaraka, Jupiter and Venus respectively, and the blemish free 7th lord and 7th house both from lagna and Moon has given a happy marriage. The aspect of Mars on Jupiter toned down by the exaltation of Saturn in a benefic sign has resulted in a headstrong but generally a pleasant married partner.

15. Female Horoscope

Though the general rules regarding the 7th house are the same for men as well as for women, still there are some special points to be observed in the female charts. This may be due to the special psycological make-up of the women. Her auspiciousness or Mangalya is read from the 8th house, issue from the 9th, beauty from the ascendant, husband and attractiveness from the 7th and association as well as chastity from the 4th house. Benefics and their lords in these houses confer good results, whereas malefics cause havoc. Some authorities hold that the lagna stands for the women's brilliance, fame and wealth, the 5th house for children and the 9th and the planets posited therein for asceticism and tranquility. If both the ascendant and moon are housed in even signs and aspected by benefics, the woman will be blessed with ideal character, prosperity, ornaments, husband and sons. If the ascendant and the moon be in odd signs and be aspected by or cojoined with malefics, she would be masculine in disposition, of crooked mind, poor, fierce and not obedient to the husband. The results would be mixed if the nature of the signs and planets be mixed.

If the 7th house or its Navamsa be a sign owned by a benefic, the woman's husband would be possessed of lustre, fame, learning and wealth provided the planets and the sign concerned are strong and unafflicted. Otherwise, he would be deformed, unintelligent, poor, deceitful or a gambler and will live away from her. If the 7th house and its amsa belong to Mars or if Mars occupies either of them she will be widowed or will be at loggerheads with the husband. She will be abandoned by her husband if there be a weak malefic in the 7th aspected by a benefic. If, on the other hand, the planets in these places are of a mixed nature, she will be remarried. Presence of malefics in the 8th house without benefic aspect will destroy the husband. However, should there be benefics in the 2nd house, the woman herself would pass away earlier.

If the 7th bhava or its navamsa belongs to a benefic the woman will have beautiful hips and be auspicious. If the trines are occupied by weak malefics, she may be either barren or will lose her children. If the Moon be posited in the 5th house identical with an Alpasutha sign (Taurus, Leo, Virgo, or Scorpio) she will have very few children. If the 7th house or its Navamsa belongs to Mars, Saturn or the Sun, her genital organ will be diseased. If the lords of the (1) ascendant, (2) the 7th, (3) 9th house and (4) the sign occupied by the Moon be posited in good houses, cojoined with benefics and be bright, the subject would be clever in doing meritorious deeds, endowed with beauty and good fortune, and respected by her kinsmen. She will be devoted to her husband, of ideal character and be blessed with good sons. The period of her sound health and auspiciousness (Mangalya) has to be read from the influence of benefics on the 8th house.

If Sun occupies the 7th house receiving the aspect of an inimical planet, she would be deserted by her husband. If Saturn be in that position receiving inimical (or malefic) aspect she would remain a spinster till the end. If the 7th house owned by a malefic be occupied by Saturn, the woman would be widowed.

When the Venus and Moon are posited in the ascendant which is owned by Mars or Saturn, and when the 5th house be also cojoined with or aspected by malefics, the woman will be barren. Similarly the Moon and Venus occupying the ascendant belonging to Mars would make the subject hate her husband; the Moon and Mercury in that position make her an expert in philosophical disquisitions; Mars and Mercury, voluptuous; the Moon, Mercury and Venus, happy and prosperous; and Jupiter blessed with good progeny, ornaments and intelligence. If the lord of the Navamsa occupied by the owner of the 8th house be malefic, widowhood is certain. If there be benefics in th

9th house, she would live happily with progeny inspite of a malefic's presence in the 7th or 8th.

When the earlier death of the woman is ascertained, the exact period of the event can be understood through the lord of the 8th house or the planet occupying it.

Nature of the Husband

When a girl's horoscope is presented for examination, you can have a fair idea as to what kind of a boy she is going to get for a husband. A few details are given below—

1. If the 7th house is devoid of strength and planets and is aspected by malefics and not by benefics, the girl will have a wretched fellow for a husband.
2. If the 7th house be occupied by Mercury and Saturn or owned by either of them, the husband will be impotent.
3. If the 7th house be a moveable sign and its lord in a moveable sign or Amsa, her husband would always be away from home.
4. If the Sun be there in his own Amsa or Sign, the husband would be gentle in his sexual activities.
5. If the Moon is similarly situated (i.e. in her own Rasi or Amsa in the 7th), he would be gentle in his sex life.
6. If it be Mars, he would be poor and adulterous.
7. If the lord is in the 9th house and Jupiter be in a Dustana (6th, 8th and 12th house) the husband would be short lived.

Hints for Ladies

Ladies have certain peculiar conditions in life. Certain ailments are peculiar to them only. First menses plays an important role in their married life. In villages a horoscope is written on this called **Ruthu Jataka**. The day and star and time of the first menses have an importance in the life of a girl.

Sunday—Less children, disease.

Monday—Good, chaste.

Tuesday—Not good for long married life.

Wednesday—Happy family.

Thursday—Happy and good character.

Friday—Healthy and devoted to husband and family.

Saturday—Vicious and short tempered.

The following stars are considered bad—Pubba, Purvabhadra, Bharani, and Aslesha. Swathi Visakha, Anuradha, Jyesta, Moola, Purvashada do not give good results as seen from Rutu-Sastra. From full or new moon day—

1. First day—virgin.
2. Beautiful.
3. Happiness.
4. Enemity.
5. Will have male children.
6. Orthodox principles.
7. Will have male issues.
8. Will lose children after delivery (of dark Moon).
9. Not happy.
10. Charitable.
11. Unhappy.
12. Healthy children.
13. Short temper.
14. Not good character.

Full or New Moon : Worker.

Certain times like sunrise and sunset, eclipse days, when some near relative expired and first month when Sun enters sign, Bharani, Krittika, Arudra, Aslesha days are bad.

Marriage is an important factor for ladies and certain combinations are very unfavourable for long, happy, married life. Mangalya Bhava from 8th, children from 5th and 9th (9th is the 5th to the 5th) regarding husband, 7th and family happiness from the 4th.

There are certain bad combinations for unhappy married life.

1. Lord of the 7th with Saturn or aspected by Mars.
2. Moon-Rahu in 8th and lord of 7th with Saturn—or Mars aspect.
3. Combination of the lords of 1 and 8 in 12 and malefic aspect on 8th.
4. Combination of the lords of 7th and 8th in 8th with malefic aspect.

Chart 1:
	Lagna		
		Mars	
	1		
		Venus	

Chart 2:
		Mars	Lagna
Moon Rahu		2	
Jupiter			

Chart 3:
	Venus Jupiter	Lagna	Mars
	3		

Chart 4:
	Mars Jupiter		
Saturn			
	4		
			Lagna

16. Health and Planets

Each sign of the Zodiac represents a certain part of the human body and the diseases peculiar to it and each planet also indicates certain types of diseases. The planetary positions at birth clearly indicate the nature of the diseases one would suffer from, when and how they would affect us and how best ot alleviate them. The 12 signs are : Aries-head; Taurus-face; Gemini-chest, arms, throat; Cancer-heart; Leo-belly; Virgo-abdominal region; Libra-lower stomach portion; Scorpio-generative organs; Sagittarius-thighs; Capricorn-knees; Aquarius-legs; Pisces-toes.

The 9 planets rule different portions of the body. In detail they are: Sun—head, eye; Moon—water, breast, glands, stomach; Mars—muscle, bile, ear, nose; Mercury—nerves, brain, spinal cord; Jupiter—Phlegm, blood; Venus—reproductive organs; Saturn—bones, joints.

The 6th house indicates the disease, 6th to 6th i.e. 11th house also indicates the nature of ailment. The planet in 6th or 11th, the combination etc and when no planet is in 6th or 11th, the aspect, received on such sign decide the nature of illness.

If the 6th Bhava is a Jalarasi and when Moon is also there, water portion of the body will be affected. When the 6th bhava is a fiery sign and when fiery planet also occupies it, danger through fire or boils are predictable.

If the 6th is an airy sign and an airy planet also occupies, the wind portion of the body will be affected, like pain in joints or excess wind in stomach. Mars indicates operation. Sun in the 6th invariably indicates hot diseases or eye troubles or headache. Mercury indicates nervousness, sleepless nights, paralysis etc. Venus gives uterus or kidney trouble, diabetes, hernia etc.

Saturn indicates pain in joints and when other factors like 8th house or 3rd house are also bad, fracture in bone etc may be the result. This planet has control over bile. Hence, jaundice or typhoid fever are also denoted.

Rahu indicates poisonous bites, mental trouble. Ketu indicates mental sickness, giddiness etc. Jupiter gives troubles in chest region like Asthma or blood sugar or blood poison, blood pressure.

Each planet is given control over some humour (dosha) causing disease and the type and seat of disease depend upon the nature of the planet and the particular sign occupied by it and the period of suffering is denoted by the Dasas and Bhuktis of such a planet as shown below:

Aries	governs	the face
Taurus	governs	the neck and the throat
Gemini	governs	upper arm and throat
Cancer	governs	breast, epigastric region and elbow
Leo	governs	back and forearm
Virgo	governs	hands and abdominal region
Libra	governs	lumbar region and loins
Scorpio	governs	external generative and urinary organs and anus
Sagittarius	governs	hips
Capricorn	governs	epidermis
Aquarius	governs	legs and ankles
Pisces	governs	toes

Precautions in predictions: The house of disease is the 6th from the Ascendant. The planets therein, the lord of the 6th, the aspects on the 6th and the navamsa, the lord of the 6th occupies, should all be considered for predicting diseases. The planets in the 6th house affect the particular part of the body governed by the sign, and the diseases will be those that are indicated by its rulers.

Due attention may be paid to the Ascendant, and the relationship between its lords and that of the 6th.

The general build-up and strength of the physical constitution must be ascertained with reference to the position of the Sun and the mental peculiarities with reference to the Moon. The Sun in the 6th aspected by saturn is sure to bring about loss of vitality by means of unnatural methods like masturbation and sodomy.

Malefics in the 6th with no beneficial aspects cause continuous illness. (Mr. X has Mercury in the 6th with Saturn and Mars powerfully aspected by Rahu—suffered from continuous artharitis for more than 25 years.)

The 8th house governs illness of a chronic type, sometimes incurable and necessitating surgey. Similarly the 12th house also beget diseases since sometimes heavy expenditure is also involved in the treatment. So all these have to be looked into. This much is enough at this stage to understand the situations. Only an expert in Medical Astrology will be able to deal the subject properly.

Some examples and case-studies are given for easy understanding.

Examples (Disease)

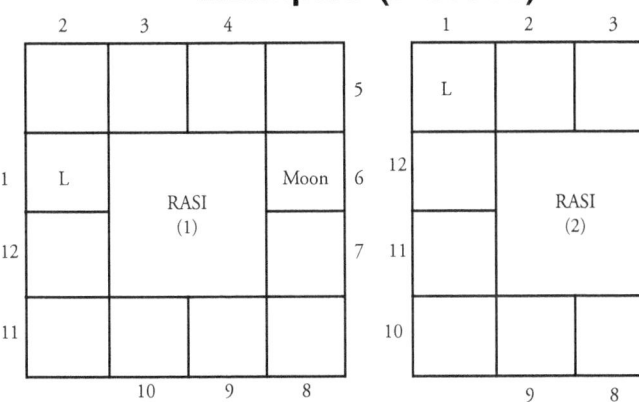

(1) Water part of the body is affected.

(2) Danger through fire or boils, eye troubles and headache.

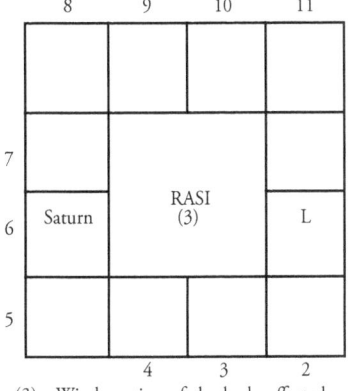

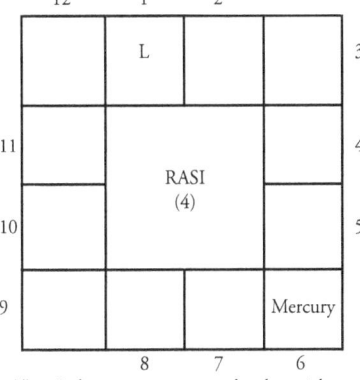

(3) Wind portion of the body affected.

(4) Indicates nervousness, sleepless nights, paralysis.

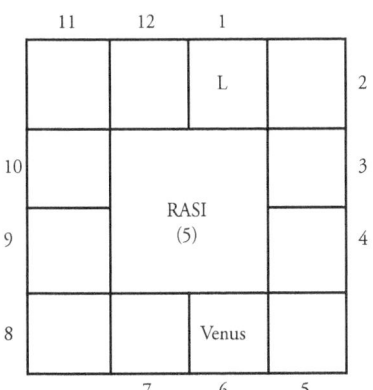

(5) Gives uterus or kidney troubles diabetes, hernia and urinary problems.

(6) Gives troubles in chest region like asthma, blood sugar, blood pressure digestive problems.

	10	11	12	
			L	1
9	RASI		2
8	(7)		3
7	Rahu		
	6	5	4	

(7) Indicates poisonous bites, mental troubles, undiagonised illness.

	7	8	9	10
	Ketu			11
	RASI		12
	(8)		
			L	
	3	2	1	

(8) Mental sickness, giddiness, Migraine, Biliouness, headache.

	10	11	12	1
			L	
9				2
8	RASI		3
	(9)		
7		Mars		
	6	5	4	

(9) Diseases due to impure blood, bone-marrow, menstrual troubles in ladies and diseases connected with head, violent tendencies, suicide tendencies.

Case-studies

	10	11	12	
		Ketu Mandi	L Jupiter	1
9	Mars Venus	RASI (1)		2
8	Sun		Saturn	3
7	Moon Mercury	Rahu		
	6	5	4	

		L Sun Saturn	Ketu Mandi
	Moon		
Jupiter		Navamsa	
Rahu Mars Mercury		Venus	

Case-1: Suffered from severe type of typhoid fever in Venus Dasa, Venus Bhukti, Saturn antara. Note Venus is in association with the lord of the 6th Mars and aspected by Saturn, lord of the 9th. Suffered from Pneumonia, loss of weight and T.B. was suspected. Also suffered from malignant malaria, pneumonia and blood vomitting.

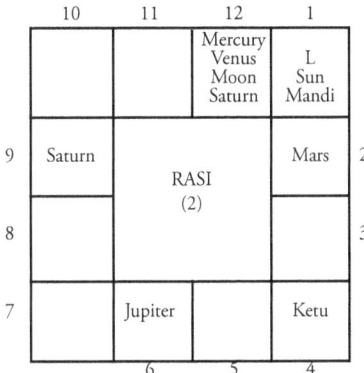

Case-2: The lord of the 6th Mars is in the 2nd (vision) and lord of the 2nd Moon (rules eye) is in the 12th with Saturn, lord of the 8th. The native suffered from Myopia.

	11	12	1	2
		Jupiter	L Sun Mercury	Venus Saturn Mandi
10		RASI (3)		Ketu	3
9	Rahu			Mars	4
8		Moon		
	7	6	5	

Venus	Rahu Jupiter Saturn Mandi	Mars	L
Sun Moon		Navamsa	
			Mercury
		Ketu	

Case-3: In Venus dasa, Rahu bhukti the native suffered severe bout of typhoid. Venus, the major lord and the lagna as well as the 6th and occupying the 2nd with saturn. Venus and Saturn are almost in conjunction. In the same dasa Saturn, Rahu he had an attack of bronchitis.

	1	2	3	4
	L	Sun Mercury		Mars Venus Jupiter
12	Rahu	RASI (4)			5
11				Ketu	6
10			Saturn	Moon
		9	8	7

Mars			Rahu
		Navamsa	
	Jupiter Moon Saturn		
Ketu	Mercury	L Sun Venus	

Case-4: The 6th is occupied by Ketu while the Moon is in Virgo subjected to serious Papakartari yoga. The 6th lord Sun is in the 2nd with Mercury, the 4th lord. The 6th from moon is occupied by Rahu and the 6th lord Saturn is in the 2nd from the Moon aspected by Sun and Mercury. The liability to attack by appendicitis is plain and unsuspectable.

	5	6	7	
	Moon			Ketu	8
4		RASI (5)			9
3				Venus Mercury Sun	10
2	Rahu	L Saturn	Jupiter	Mars	
	1	12	11	

	Mercury Venus	Rahu	Sun Mars
Jupiter Saturn		Navamsa	
	Ketu		L Moon

Case-5: Is the horoscope of a lady and she was troubled by paralysis of the lower limbs and arms. The 6th is Aries and is aspected by Mars being lord of that house. The 6th from moon has the Sun (lord of 6th with Venus) (lord of 3rd and 8th) and Mercury rules nerves aspected by Saturn. These attributes denote the disposition of the house of disease. 9th house rules the limbs. Here the 9th from the Moon is Scorpio and the 9th lord Mars aspects Moon. The 9th is occupied by Saturn, a first rate malefic. Saturn is the planet of obstruction. Thus the whole region of the lower limbs is affected.

17. Profession

As you are aware the 10th house is called the house of profession or Karma, which forms the very foundation, as it were, of the edifice of human life. Profession forms one of the most fundamental factors of man's mundane life. Accordingly the 10th house is called as the Meridian, highest point.

Students of astrology are aware that the general method of reading a person's profession is through the lord of the Navamsa occupied by the lord of 10th house. But this is not an infallible method. There are many other factors which go into the making of profession. Man follows some vocation because he likes it and through that he wishes to earn his livelihood. If one gets good deal of honour and wealth from his profession, he is said to have a good and comfortable position/profession. There are several grades of professional status. One may become a menial, another a clerk, yet another a minister and so on.

First of all we have to consider the Ascendant, its lord aspects and planets posted in it. For, the first Bhava represents the Body with which we have to perform all our actions. Then the position and strength of the Moon also have to be taken into consideration. The moon is born of the mind of the creator. Then we have to note the strength and position of the Sun who is the soul of the Universe. The strength and good position of the benefics also are essential for ensuring a good and happy life. Benefics should generally occupy in strength Kendras and malefics the 3rd, 6th and 11th receiving benefic aspects. It is also more important that benefics should generally be more powerful than malefics. But the lord of Bhagya-fortune-whoever might be, must be strong, well-aspected and well-situated. The lord of Karma too must be similarly placed in a Kona, which is atleast a friendly house. It is better there is connection between the lords of the Lagna, Bhagya, and Karma. Similarly the lords of wealth and gain (2nd and 11th) among others must be strong and well placed. The same remark applies to the lords of happiness and intelligence (4th and 5th). If all these conditions are satisfied, the subject is sure to occupy a high position of honour, getting plenty of money and homage. He will also discharge his duties efficiently and honourably.

Infact, when you consider a particular Bhava, all the other Bhavas also come into the picture in some relationship or the other, as they are all intrinsically connected with it. For example, the 6th house becomes the 10th from the house of fortune. Hence, no Bhava examined in isolation could give an accurate account of itself. It is not these Bhavas and their lords alone that give us a clue to a man's position, mode of life and activities. There are certain positions of planets in the Signs of the Zodiac and Yogas which at once tell you whether the subject is a prince or peasant, wealthy or bankrupt, physician or patient, and so on. If Jupiter be posted in the 8th house, the native would be poor and earn his living as a menial. On the other hand, if Jupiter should be in the 9th, he could aspire to become a minister. So too Venus occupying the 2nd house makes one a poet and wealthy. The same planet in the 10th enables one to have a comfortable position. Saturn in the lagna identical with his own or exaltation sign produces one equal to a king, or a mayor. But in the several lagnas indicates some sort of professional leanings. For example one born in Vrishabha lagna would be engaged in agriculture. One born in Mithuna could read other's thoughts or becomes a psychologist and take interest in dancing and music. Birth in Virgo gives the power of interpreting sastras or scriptures. Libra makes one clever in trade, Scorpio a Govt. servant or an employer in a palace, Capricorn a religious hypocrite. Similarly different constellations produce different learnings.

The existence of excellent Yogas like Mahayogas,

Rajayogas, Mahapurusha yogas, Mahabhagya, Kesari, Adhiyoga, Vasumati Puskala, Lakshmi, Saraswati etc. contribute to great fortune, eminence and certain professional bias. All these things drive us to conclude that the whole horoscope should be judged as a single unit and its status ascertained before venturing a prediction. Conjunction of planets also give some clues to professional tendencies.

Many a time the planets occupying or aspecting the Ascendant contribute their qualities for the formation of vocation. Still the most common and popular method is to read the profession from the lord of the Navamsa occupied by the lord of the 10th house counted from the strongest of the three viz. Ascendant, Moon and Sun. But in my opinion it is always better to consider from the Ascendant itself and not others. Regarding the 10th house too there are several factors to be taken into consideration: (1) Lord of the Bhava, (2) Lord of the Sign occupied by the lord of the 10th, (3) Planets in the 10th house, (4) Planets aspecting the 10th, (5) Lord of the Navamsa occupied by the 10th lord. All these planets or the strongest of them will contribute the share to formulate the Native's profession. In all cases, if the planet concerned be very strong, the subject would be able to earn wealth without much effort and be quite happy. Otherwise the result will vary according to the planet's strength. If the Sign mentioned above is occupied or aspected by its own lord, the person will earn his living in his own country. On the otherhand, if the planet owning the Rasi or Amsa is in a moveable sign, he will earn money in a foreign country. If the said lord is retrograde, he will earn money from various sources. But one's measure of wealth entirely depends on one's fortune—9th house and its lord etc. A single benefic in the 10th from Moon or Lagna without contact with or aspect of inimical planets will usher into the world a person enjoying the company of a large family and everlasting fame.

The planet and the sign show a broad outline of the nature of profession in modern days. When Science is said to be advancing, branches of studies are increasing. In a period of 40 years, 1940-80 we can know the various new branches and many old branches subdivided and so on.

Similarly in securing a job also the line of education and the nature of job have little bearing; to cite an example, a Zoology postgraduate getting a job in Bank or Postoffice. The planets do give a broad outline even if more branches are forthcoming.

Sun: Authority, dealing in precious metals, dealing in money, bank etc. Compared to present itmes branches of study are I.A.S. B.Com, M.A., M.Com, M.Sc., etc.

Moon: (Water, which travels from place to place in the form of cloud.) Travelling salesman, Navy, fishing, water as base, mild vending or milk products. Moon is attached to human mind. Hence, imagination in writing or poetic.

Branches more suitable are M.Sc., Chemistry, Journalism Navy Engineering.

Mars: (Blood red) poisonous gases, engineering operations, Surgeon, Police etc. Branches are Engineering branches, Medical Laboratories, M.Tech, A.M.I.E., B.E., M.D. or M.B.B.S., I.P.S.

Mercury: This is the business magnet. Stock exchange, Publication, Printing, Travel, Branches are B.A., (Ecom) B.Com. Journalism, Banking Exams, M.Sc. (Maths) I.F.S.

Jupiter: What one learns has to be given to others (priest). From elementary school teacher to that of Reader in University is the field of Jupiter. Politics is also an apt field. Religion is born. Hence position as Trustee of a temple is also suitable. Branches are M.A., M.Lit, in any language, learning veda, M.A. Politics, M.A. Philosophy.

Venus: This stands for luxury, and less physical effort. Dealing in cloth, silks, precious stones, diamond setters, sale of readymade garments etc. Venus stands for art also. Music, drawing, photography, painting etc.

Generally drawing and music comes by nature from tender age. When this art is seen, it will be wise to give them training in that field.

Saturn: This is a slow moving planet. Patience is required for certain studies. Saturn stands for authority also. He controls over iron and oil.

Hence, the branches are M.Sc. (Maths), or Doctorate or Research field, Electrical Engineering, Aeroplane Engineering, Auto engineering etc. Dealing in iron and hardware, oil mill etc., are also suitable.

Rahu: This stands for engineering, inflammable gases and politics. Branches are M.Tech, B.E., M.A. Politics.

Ketu: Religion and art appeal more. M.A., Philosophy, photography, religious preachers etc., are better, suitable lines.

The 10th place is Jivanasthana. The planet in the 10th Bhava decides the nature of profession. The lord of the 10th also decides this, the sign of the 10th also decides this.

For example, if Cancer is 10th and Moon in Cancer Chemistry, Botany, Agriculture, dealing in liquids etc. are apt. If Leo happens to be in the 10th place and when Sun is there, Govt. position is likely.

18. Gochara (Transit)

The word Gochara simply means movement of planets along the circle of Zodiac. You have already seen how a planet produces effects, good or bad, during its Dasa. This Dasa-mythology is based upon the natal chart as a whole. The Gochara system, however, is based upon the transit or movement of planets from time to time through the various Sign of the Zodiac starting, of course, from a fixed point viz: the position of the Natal Moon. No doubt, there are important factors in a horoscope viz. the Ascendant, the Moon's sign and one occupied by the Sun. So the effects of transit must be considered with reference to all these three factors. Still the ancients have given greater weight and consideration to the Moon's position at birth. The reason for this is not far to seek. For, the Moon is the Cosmic Mind or the one born of the mind of the Supreme. When such is the case, it is but right that the Moon should be considered as the pivot for the changing fortunes of all beings. Moreover, in the Gochara system generally the planets as such are considered and not as owners of Bhavas. Now the details of the Gochara system are given. Taking the natal Moon as the starting point you have to proceed to consider which planets are good or bad and in which houses.

The Sun produces the good effects when he passes in transit through the 3rd, 6th, 10th and 11th houses from the Moon. The moon is beneficial in 1, 3, 6, 7, 10 and 11 places from herself. Mercury is auspicious in 2, 4, 6, 8, 10 and 11 places from the Moon. Jupiter is good in 2, 5, 7, 9 and 11 places. Venus is favourable in 1, 2, 3, 4, 5, 8, 9, 11 and 12 places. Generally the nine planets beginning with the Sun take respectively the following periods to pass through a rasi (1) one month, (2) 2 days, (3) 1½ months,

(4) 1 month, (5) one year (6) 1 month (7) 2 ½ years (8) and (9) 1 ½ years. Though a planet is expected to produce its effects good or bad, throughout the period of its passage over a house, still has a particular part of that period which is considered most potent. They are respectively for the planets beginning with the Sun (1) the first 5 days, (2) the last 3 ghatis, (3) the first 8 days (4) throughout the period of 1 month, (5) 2 months in the middle (6) 7 days in the middle (7) the last six months, (8) & (9) the last 3 months. The same may be put in another form as follows—The Sun and Mars produce effects when they pass through the initial 10 degrees of a Rasi, Jupiter and Venus in the middle 10 degrees, the Moon and Saturn in the last 10 degrees and Mercury and Rahu throughout their passage.

There is another term called Vedha, which means 'piercing' which means 'undoing' or 'cancellation'. For every place producing good or bad effects there is a place called Vedha which when occupied by some other planet nullifies the previous effects. For example, the Sun is good in transit when he passes through the 3rd house but its Vedha is the 9th house. The idea is though Sun is transiting the 3rd house from the Natal Moon, should yield very good results, still there would be nothing good coming out of this position, if at that time some planet (other than Saturn) transits the 9th house from the Moon. In the same manner bad effects too are nullified by their Vedha positions being tenanted by some other planets at the same time. The following are the Vedha positions of all the planets:

The denominator figure given below each nominator figure is the Vedhanka (point of obstruction) for it:

Sun: $\dfrac{11\text{-}3\text{-}10\text{-}6}{5\text{-}9\text{-}4\text{-}12}$

Moon: $\dfrac{7\text{-}1\text{-}6\text{-}11\text{-}10\text{-}3}{2\text{-}5\text{-}12\text{-}8\text{-}4\text{-}9}$

Mars: $\dfrac{3\text{-}11\text{-}6}{12\text{-}5\text{-}9}$

Mercury: $\frac{2-4-6-8-10-11}{5-3-9-1-7-12}$

Jupiter: $\frac{2-11-9-5-7}{12-8-10-4-3}$

Venus: $\frac{1-2-3-4-5-8-9-11-12}{8-7-10-9-5-11-6-3}$

Saturn: $\frac{3-11-6}{12-5-9}$

Gochara and Dasa Bhukti go side by side. A Dasa may be bad, Gochara may be good to rectify the bad.

A Dasa may be very good but the transit Saturn in Janam Rasi as 7½ years period gives bad results. In many cases both agree to do major good or both disagree to neutralise or both plan to give a major calamity. In deciding gochara there are certain basic principles. The Gochara of Jupiter decides the course for an year and Saturn for 2 ½ years. It is fitting to state that Jupiter-Saturn are makers of destiny.

Each star has its own favourable and unfavourable position. They are grouped as Janma, Anujanma or Trijanma stars in the order of 2, 4, 6, 8, 9 from birth star are favourable while stars 3, 5, 7 are bad.

(1) Janma (2) Sampath - Prosperity (3) Vipath - adversity (4) Kshema - welfare (5) Prytayak - failure (6) Sadhana -favourable (7) Naidhana (vadham) - fight (8) Maitram -friendship (9) Parama Mitra very friendly.

Thus the stars or constellations in 3-5-7 from Janma Nakshatra star are unfavourable. Suppose the janma star is Aswini, let us see how they reflect.

The 10th star from the birth star is known as Trikona. Thus for Aswini the Trikona is Makham and from Makham it is Moola. 2, 4, 6, 8 stars together with Trikona gives good in their respective Dasa Bhukti or their position in Gochara also.

The 3-5-7 from Janma or Anujanma or Trijanma are not

favourable stars. The movement of the planets are noted in reference to the stars. A planet may be seen in a particular sign at a given time. But the star position may be different, since 2 stars are for a sign. Take for example a man born in the 5th sign, favourable results are to be seen. This 5th house is Leo. This has Makah, Pubba and Uttars 1st part.

Suppose Jupiter is in Uttara star, this is in the 3rd place from Anujanma which is Vipat Tara. Instead of favourable result, opposite results will be realised.

Thus a planet to give good results has two basic requirements. His position as Trikona or Kendra etc. His star position as Sampath or Vipat or Kshema or Naidhana (Vadham).

Since the Gochara of Jupiter for 1 year and saturn for 2½ years play major role than others which move more quickly. Let us see the results in detail:

SUN

1. Janma Rasi: Loss of prestige and money, ill health, wandering.
2. Fear, anxiety, more work and less income.
3. New status, observing Dharma, happiness and joy.
4. Litigation, quarrel, disease.
5. Disease, official displeasure, separation from son or other relatives.
6. Recoupment of health, victory, cheer, fame and success.
7. Stomach disorder, journey, fear anxiety.
8. Even wife will not be happy, sorrow, disease to son or wife.
9. Quarrel on account of money, despair.
10. Success in business or honour in work place, good health, financial improvement.
11. Success and higher position, prosperity and good health.
12. Sorrow, quarrel, ill health.

Sun is thus favourable in 3, 6, 10, 11. Sun is in one sign

for a month. Hence, his position is the nature of event for a month.

MOON

1. Good food, jolly mood.
2. Loss and obstacles.
3. Wealth and victory.
4. Mental worry, uneasiness.
5. Obstacles and sorrow.
6. Victory, good health.
7. Conveyance, good food, no financial anxiety.
8. Misery, ill health (This is known as Chandrastama. Generally these 2 days, 3 days is a trying period.)
9. Anxiety, upset of stomach.
10. Position and success.
11. Meeting new friends, happiness.
12. Loss, mental anxiety.

Moon is good in 1, 3, 6, 7, 10, 11.

MARS

1. Trouble from superiors, displeasure, loss of money, obstacles.
2. Quarrels, disputes, excess bile and ill health.
3. New position of authority, financial betterment, gain, good health.
4. Fever, disease of blood or stomach, loss of character.
5. More enemies, trouble from son, loss of energy.
6. Victory over enemies, relief from troubles, independence, wealth and cheer.
7. Quarrel with wife, upset of stomach, vain attempts, cares and anxieties.
8. Poison, more worries, dependence.
9. Wounds from instruments, aimless journey.
10. Mixed events.

11. Gain, new position.
12. Quarrel, excitement, trouble through ladies.
    Hence, Mars is good in 3, 6, 11.

MERCURY

1. Loss of money due to wrong advice of ladies and friends.
2. Digrace, dishonour, some money and success.
3. Friends, afraid of troubles due to Royal displeasure.
4. Gain of money, family happiness.
5. Separation from son and wife, no enjoyment.
6. Victory, happiness, higher status.
7. Misery, anxiety, quarrel, less bright in outlook.
8. Victory, gain, happiness through son, new clothes.
9. Upset of health and obstacles.
10. Victory over enemies, gets wealth, enjoys lady's company.
11. Comforts from son, money and enjoyment, mental peace.
12. Troublesome journeys, disgrace.
    Thus Mercury is good in 4, 6, 8, 10, 11 positions.

JUPITER

1. Loss of place or position and wealth, quarrel and mental tension.
2. Gain of wealth and enjoyment of money and women.
3. Trouble due to loss of property, despair, mental agony.
4. Trouble from relations, despair, loss, lowering of status, obstacles.
5. Gain, servants, marriage or auspicious ceremonies, improvement in education, noble qualities, clothes, prosperity.
6. Quarrel with relatives, anxiety, fear and failure in activities.
7. Good food and drink, cheer, expansion of knowledge,

company of excellent women, conveyance and wealth.
8. Death, disgrace, danger or serious illness, travel giving much fatigue.
9. Birth of child, marriage, new status, honour, wealth, much influence, income from gain and grocery shop.
10. Change in place of work, transfer, loss of health and money due to suffering from phlegm etc.
11. Recovery from disease, gain from son, enjoys women, wealth, vehicle.
12. Travel to distant place, anxiety, mental tension.

Jupiter is good in 2, 5, 7, 9, 11 position.

VENUS

1. Good food, enjoyments of women, comfort in bedding.
2. Gain of wealth, Royal honour and happiness.
3. Influence, new status, prestige.
4. New friends, power, honour.
5. Happiness, birth of son, auspicious ceremonies at home, fame and wealth.
6. Disgrace, disease, quarrel.
7. Evils through ladies, gain from wicked people.
8. Sexual happiness, honour, clothes and building houses.
9. Virtuous, happiness, good children and wealthy.
10. Disgrace, quarrel, even when measured words in talk will bring disputes or misunderstanding.
11. Wealth from friends, good food, perfumes and happiness.
12. Gain of money but loss of clothes.

Venus is good in 1, 2, 3, 4, 5, 8, 9, 11, 12.

SATURN

The gochara of saturn is very important and decides the general trend of events of 2½ years. When Saturn transits in 12, 1, 2, position of Moon, it is known as 7½ years Saturn period i.e. Sadesathe. Normally there are two such occasions assuming the span as 60 and more. It plays a key role in the career. It is not correct to say that the individual will suffer for full 7½ years.

Suppose there is serious illness for one or two months, this is enough to give extra medical bill, extra expense to recoup lost health, displeasure in office due to absence and the like. The individual has to bear this loss for a long period to become normal.

Suppose in a family, wife, son or daughter may all have the same janma rasi and this may give 7½ years saturn period to all. In this case it is not quite encouraging. Suffering is seen in turn.

Suppose they have different Rasis when the wife is having 7½ year period, this affects husband also indirectly since he is the head of the family. If the marriageable daughter is having this Saturn period her marriage may be delayed and the parents will have mental worry.

Hence, in a family some member has this influence. Prevention is better than cure. Before the beginning of this period set apart $1/10$ of your monthly income to Annadanam.

This is not merely giving a few coins to a roadside beggar but rice preparations of some kichidi or kheer at home and distribution to the beggars with sincerity. Serious illness during this period can be avoided by this way.

Practical experience will reveal this. Even when disease comes it will pass off easily. A wound may be small caused by a blade when the pencil is sharpened or from a car. Fate is there but the velocity can be minimised.

1. Loss of house, separation from wife and children, leaves his place, suffering caused by fire or poison, travel on foot.
2. Loss of beauty, no comfort, weakness and expenses.
3. Prosperity, wealth and enjoyment, servant's influence, power, recovery from disease, victory over enemies.
4. Separation from family, loss of status or position, suspicion in everything, loss of wealth.
5. Separation from son, loss of wealth, many disputes,

court troubles.
6. Victory over enemies, company of women, improvement in finance.
7. Disease in generative organ, separation from wife and children, pitiable conditions.
8. Mental worry, journey, weakness, hunger, does mean actions.
9. Much suffering and will not do even his religious duties, suffer from enemity, cases or imprisonment.
10. Vast learning and fame but financial loss.
11. Cruel mind, will get some comfort from fair sex or wealth.
12. Much grief, calamities.

Hence, Saturn is good in 3, 6, 11 (to some extent) Rahu takes the qualities of Saturn and Ketu that of Mars.

To decide the gochara result a very critical study is required. Jupiter may be in the 5th house but Saturn will be in the Janma Rasi in 7 ½ years round. Or Jupiter may be in 12 and a turn may be in 6th. Thus good is neutralised by bad as seen at a glance. But in reality it may not be so. Jupiter in the 5th house if in bad tara may not give good and similarly if Saturn is in good Tara may not give bad. The whole is a complicated one and patient study is necessary to decide the course. The other quick moving planets except Rahu, Ketu change their influence often.

A chart for easy reference is given to know the position at a glance.

Planet	Good position	Bad position
Sun	3, 6, 10, 11	1, 2, 4, 5, 7, 8, 9. 12
Moon	1, 3, 6, 7, 10, 11	2, 4, 5, 8, 9, 12
Mars	3, 6, 11	1, 2, 4, 5, 7, 8, 9, 10, 12
Jupiter	2, 5, 7, 9, 11	1, 3, 4, 6, 8, 10,12

Mercury	2, 4, 6, 8, 10, 11		1, 3, 6, 7, 9, 12
Venus	1,2,3,4,5,8,9,11,12		6, 7, 10
Saturn	3, 6, 11		1, 2, 4, 5, 7, 8, 9, 10, 12

	Janma	**Anujanma**	**Trijanma**
	1. Aswini	10. Makham	19. Moola
Sampath	2. Bharani	11. Pubba	20. Purvashada
Vipat	3. Krithika	12. Uttara	21. Uttarashada
Kshemam	4. Rohini	13. Hastha	22. Sravana
Prytyak	5. Mrigasira	14. Chitta	23. Dhanista
Sadhana	6. Aridra	15. Swathi	24. Satabhisha
Naidhana	7. Punarvasu	16. Visaka	25. Purvabhadra
Mitra	8. Pushyami	17. Anuradha	26. Uttarabhadra
Parama Mitra	9. Aslesha	18. Jyesta	27. Revathi.

19. Hora

Among the various factors that strengthen an event, Hora is one important factor. A day has a force of planet and the day is divided to seven divisions/cycle and each division is ruled by a planet. There is an order behind this.

For each day the rising planet of that day is Sun for Sunday, Moon for Monday, Mars for Tuesday, Mercury for Wednesday, Jupiter for Thursday, Venus for Friday and Saturn for Saturday. The house is worked from sunrise. A chart is appended. For benefic activities specific Hora will bring benefic results.

Sun Hora: Interview, for posting applications for appointment, all dealings with the Govt. or superiors in authority.

Moon Hora: Mental work, writing articles or stories, writing important letters, dealings in liquids, attending to matters relating to ladies.

Mars Hora: Land operations, instrument work, or weapons etc. Generally it is preferable to think well and talk or offer opinions or otherwise unnecessary quarrel may cause.

Mercury Hora: All kinds of business activities, writing work, selling old articles of home will fetch more money.

Jupiter Hora: Prayers, agriculture, seeing persons of authority, applying for job, marriage talks or other auspicious functions, learning new fields of education, learning music and Veda.

Venus Hora: Prayers, marriage talks, purchasing ornaments or clothes, to raise loan or discharge loan.

Saturn Hora: Dealing with iron or hardware, agriculture operations, taking medicines.

We have seen the importance of the lords of 5, 9, and 10. The hora relating to them may also be selected with advantage. The chart is as follows:

Hour	Sun	Mon	Tues	Wed	Thurs	Friday	Sat
6-7	Sun	Moon	Mars	Mercury	Jupiter	Venus	Saturn
7-8	Venus	Saturn	Sun	Moon	Mars	Mercury	Jupiter
8-9	Mercury	Jupiter	Venus	Saturn	Sun	Moon	Mars
9-10	Moon	Mars	Mercury	Jupiter	Venus	Saturn	Sun
10-11	Saturn	Sun	Moon	Mars	Mercury	Jupiter	Venus
11-12	Jupiter	Venus	Saturn	Sun	Moon	Mars	Mercury
12-1	Mars	Mercury	Jupiter	Venus	Saturn	Sun	Moon
1-2	Sun	Moon	Mars	Mercury	Jupiter	Venus	Sat
2-3	Venus	Saturn	Sun	Moon	Mars	Mercury	Jupiter
3-4	Mercury	Jupt	Venus	Saturn	Sun	Moon	Mars
4-5	Moon	Mars	Mercury	Jupiter	Venus	Sat	Sun
5-6	Saturn	Sun	Moon	Mars	Mercury	Jupt	Venus
6-7	Jupt	Venus	Saturn	Sun	Moon	Mars	Mercury
7-8	Mars	Mercury	Jupiter	Venus	Sat	Sun	Moon
8-9	Sun	Moon	Mars	Mercury	Jupt	Venus	Saturn
9-10	Venus	Saturn	Sun	Moon	Mars	Mercury	Jupiter
10-11	Mercury	Jupt	Venus	Saturn	Sun	Moon	Mars
11-12	Moon	Mars	Mercury	Jupiter	Venus	Sat	Sun
12-1	Saturn	Sun	Moon	Mars	Mercury	Jupt	Venus
1-2	Jupiter	Venus	Saturn	Sun	Moon	Mars	Mercury
2-3	Mars	Mercury	Jupiter	Venus	Saturn	Sun	Moon
3-4	Sun	Moon	Mars	Mercury	Jupt	Venus	Saturn
4-5	Venus	Saturn	Sun	Moon	Mars	Mercury	Jupiter
5-6	Mercury	Jupiter	Venus	Saturn	Sun	Moon	Mars

The middle portion of the Hora has greater force.

20. Death

Nobody knows about the soul before its incarnation as well as after its disincarnation. During this interval it plays a wonderful role on the stage of life. Hence, both the initial and final points of its life assume unusual importance.

You are aware that the house concerned with the death is the 8th. So are the planets that are connected with this house. If the 8th house is neither occupied nor aspected by planets, then death could be expected as a result of the special nature of humour of the sign representing the 8th house, or of the Navamsa Sign occupied by the lord of the 8th. The following are the effects of the 12 houses beginning with Aries, happening to be the 8th house or the Amsa of its lord:

Aries: Death will be due to fever, poison, stomach disease and billiouness.

Taurus: It is due to the vitiation of all the humours, weapons or fire.

Gemini: It is caused by cough, asthma, excessive heat, colic etc.

Cancer: It is through rheaumatism, insanity or diarrhoea.

Leo: It is due to boils (Tumour), poison, weapons, fever etc.

Virgo: It is through stomach complaints, disease of the private parts, quarrel, fall from a precipice etc.

Libra: It is caused by aberration of mind, fever or typhoid.

Scorpio: Through jaundice, diarrhoea, enlargement of the spleen and the like.

Sagittarius: Through a tree, water, weapon or wooden piece. (The effect is sure if the concerned sign of amsa is occupied by the malefic).

Capricorn: It is by impalement, ploughing or mental derangement. If there is a malefic in the Sign or Amsa, death is likely through wild animals, tigers, cough, fever, consumption or some unnatural cause.

Aquarius: If it is occupied by malefics, death is likely through tigers, weapons, serpents, cough, fever or consumption.

Pisces: It may be due to snake-poison, exhaustion of a journey, storm, machine, shipwreck or fall of lightning.

In case 8th house is occupied by any one of the seven planets beginning with Sun, the end may be brought about by (1) fire, (2) water, (3) weapon, (4) fall, (5) fever, (6) thirst or diabetes, and (7) starvation in that order.

On the other hand if this house is aspected by strong planets, the cause of the death may be the particular humours belonging to them. Now we can also know if the subject is going to die in his own house or away from one's house or abroad. If the 8th house is a moveable sign, death will take place in a foreign country, if it is a fixed one, at home, and if a dual one, on the way or near home.

If the ascendant is a Nocturnal sign, death will occur at night and if Diurnal at day time. It is understood that if there are planets in the Lagna, they would influenced the effects.

One dies with many others, if there are many planets in the 4th, and the lord of the ascendant is cojoined with that of the 8th house.

One would die along with one's wife or son, if the lords of the ascendant and the 8th house are cojoined with that of the 7th or 5th house, as the case may be.

If the lord of Lagna be in a watery sign or Amsa being aspected by the Moon and Venus, and if the 8th and 12th houses are occupied by malefics, death will be in water.

If the birth takes place during the period of Visha Ghatis and if the 8th house be occupied by a malefic, death would be through poison, fire or weapons.

If the Moon be in the fatal degrees in the Ascendant, 8th or 12th house, it would be through water or machinery.

If the lord of the 8th house be posted in a Navamsa which is termed Visha, and be cojoined with a malefic, death would be by snake poison, by vultures or by wild boars according to the name of the particular Navamsa.

The first Navamsa of Aries, Taurus, Virgo and Sagittarius the middle of Gemini, Leo, Libra and Aquarius, and the last of the Cancer, Scorpio, Capricorn and Pisces are respectively called, Snake-poison, Vulture poison and Boar-poison.

A few examples and case-studies are given for clear understanding.

Examples (Death)

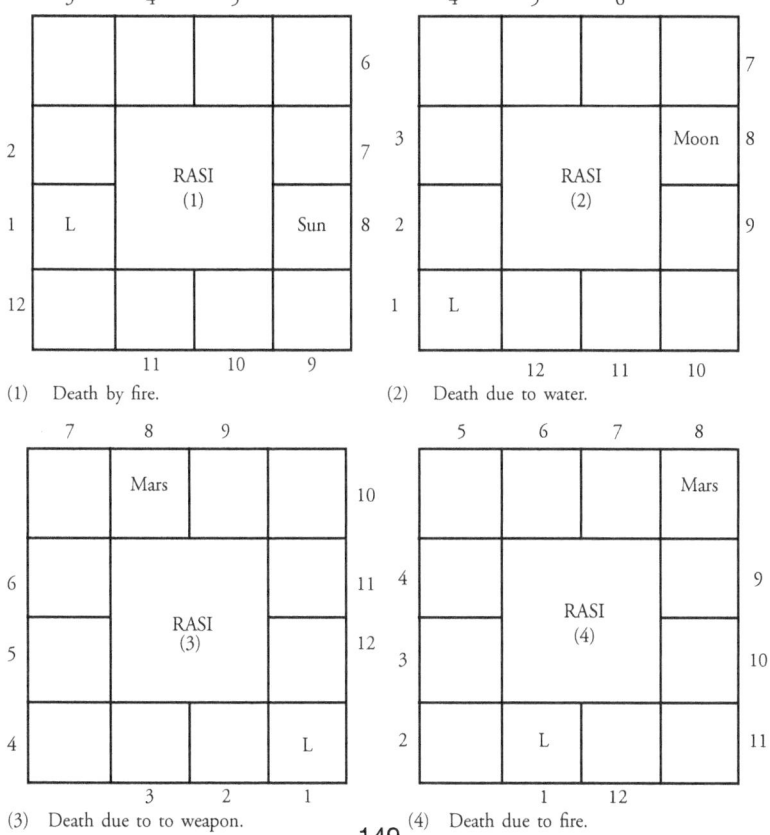

(1) Death by fire.
(2) Death due to water.
(3) Death due to to weapon.
(4) Death due to fire.

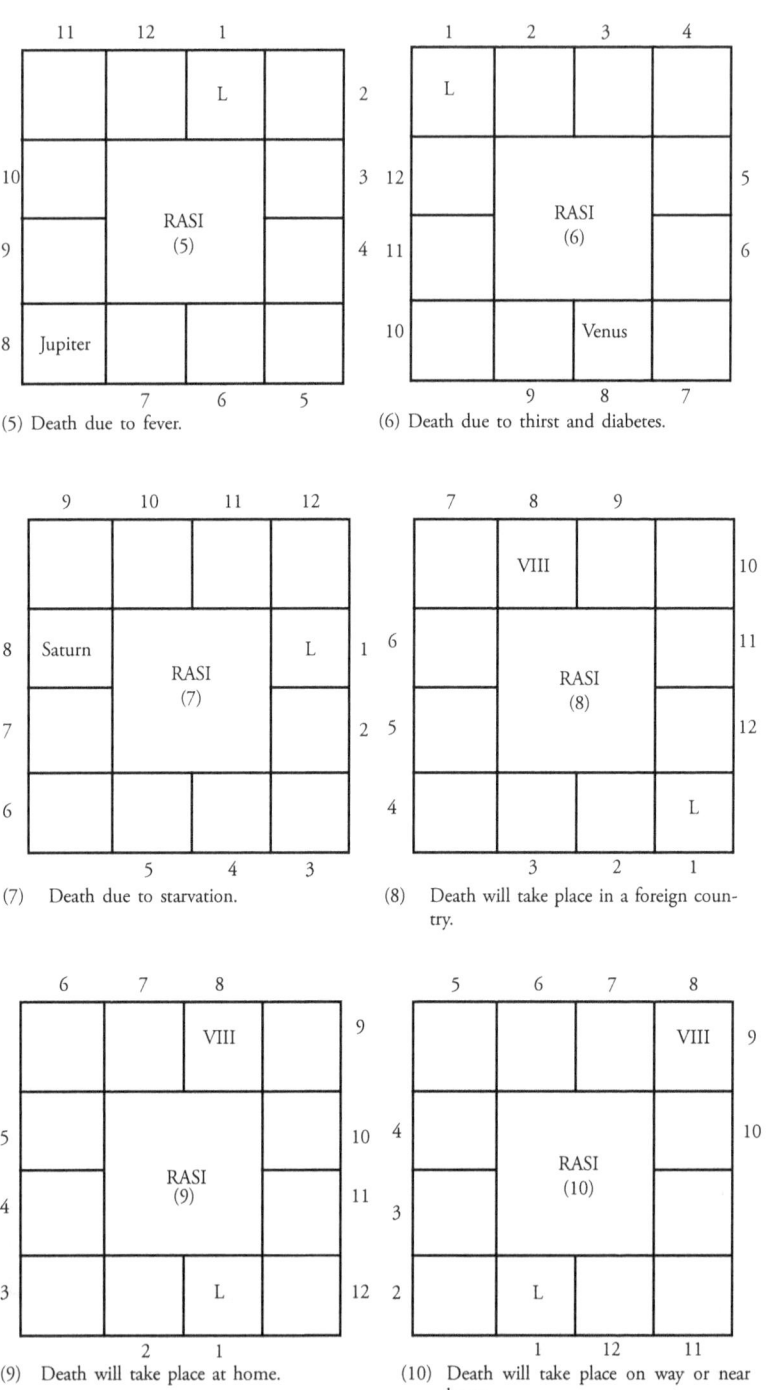

(5) Death due to fever.

(6) Death due to thirst and diabetes.

(7) Death due to starvation.

(8) Death will take place in a foreign country.

(9) Death will take place at home.

(10) Death will take place on way or near home.

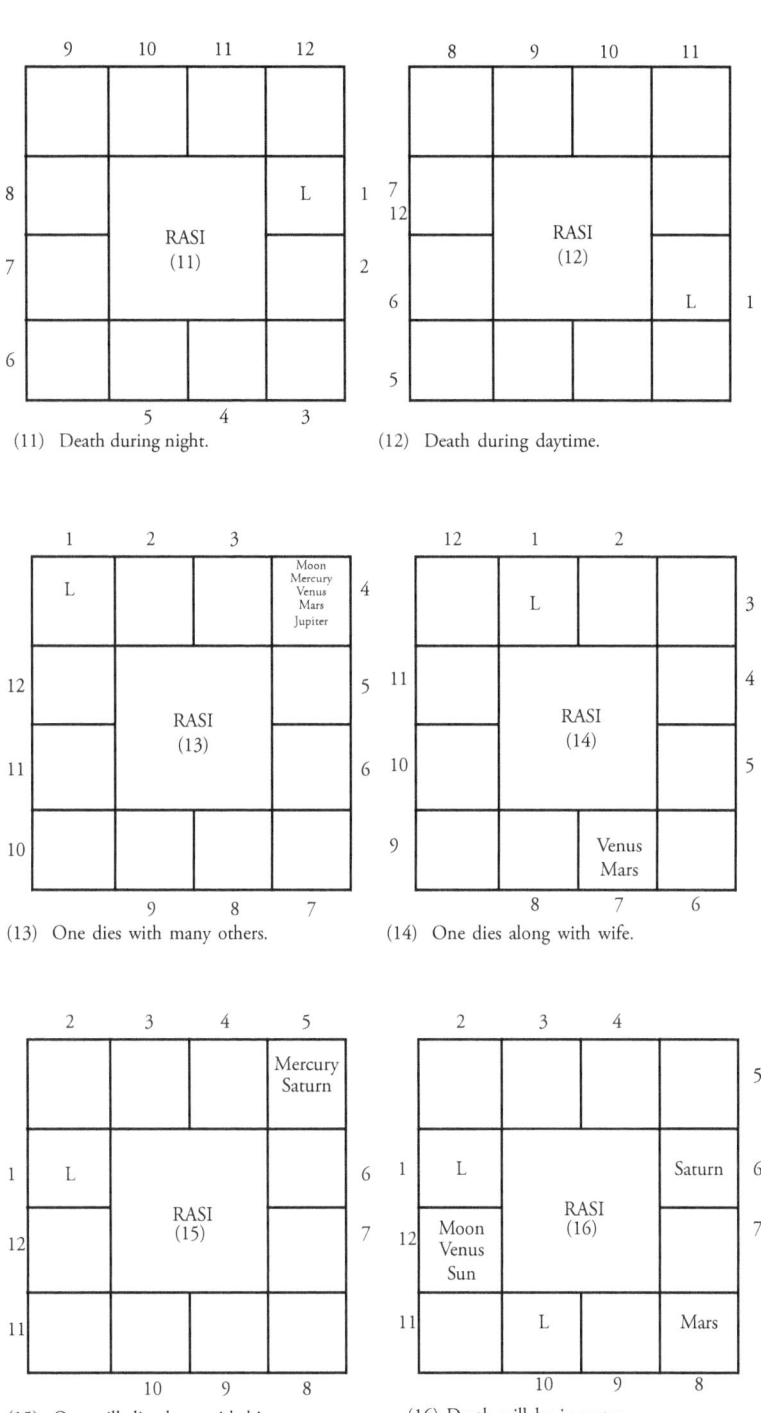

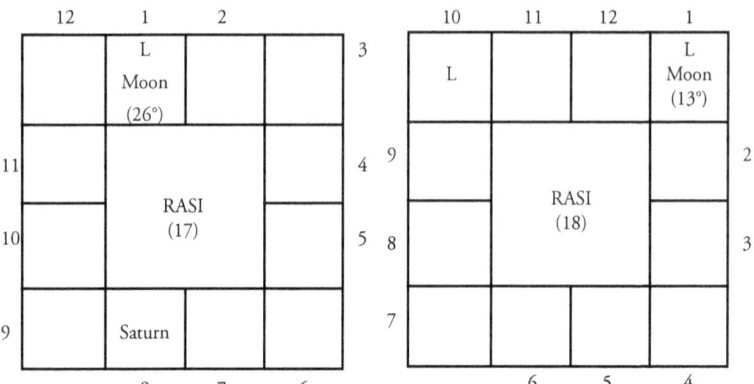

(17) Death will be due to poison, fire a weapon.

(18) Death will be due to water machinery

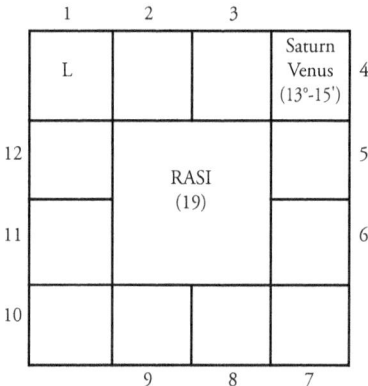

(19) Death will be due to snake poison.

Case-studies

		Jupiter	Moon Rahu	11
Venus	RASI (1)			12
Sun			L	1
Mercury Saturn Ketu			Mars	

Moon Rahu	L	Mars	
	Navamsa		Sun
			Jupiter Saturn
Mercury	Venus		Ketu

1. A case of Balarista: The Moon is afflicated by Rahu and Saturn. He does not receive any benefic aspects. Both Moon and Rahu move into the 12th Bhava. The Child died within 3 years.

	Ketu		Moon		
		RASI (2)		L	1
	Saturn			Venus	2
		Jupiter	Sun Mars	Rahu Mercury	

Moon	Rahu Saturn	Mars	
	Navamsa		L
			Mercury
Venus Mars	Sun	Ketu Jupiter	

2. A case of Alpayu: The Ascendant and the 8th house and their lords are weak either due to occupation, aspect, or other afflictions. Benefics are also weak while malefics may be strong in the kendras. The lagna is fairly strong being Vargottama and lagna lord is exalted in an asterism of the 2nd lord Sun. Strong malefics occupy kendras. Saturn aspects the Lagna adversely. 3rd house and the 2nd lord are both afflicted by Rahu and Mars and Saturn. The Native died at 16 years in Ketu Bhukti, Mars Dasa.

Rasi (3)

		Moon Jupiter	Ketu
	RASI (3)		Saturn
Venus			
Mercury Sun Rahu			L Mars

Houses: 7, 8, 9, 10 (top); 11, 12 (right); 3, 2, 1 (bottom); 6, 5, 4 (left)

Navamsa

	L Moon Jupiter		
Mars			Rahu Sun
Saturn Ketu	Navamsa		
Mercury			Venus

3. A case of Madhyayu: Lagna lord is in a kendra afflicted and eclipsed. 8th lord too is in kendra aspected by the 7th lord Jupiter. But Jupiter occupies the asterism of a benefic Moon. So also Saturn occupies the constellation of Lagna Lord. Here both malefics and benefics occupy trines and quadrants indicating medium life. Also this is a yoga. If the 8th lord is in a kendra and 8th house is not occupied by any planets the Native lives for 40 years:

Death took place in Mercury Bhukti, Jupiter Dasa. Jupiter is the 7th lord from Lagna and hence a killer. Mercury being lagna lord is highly afflicted and becomes a maraka.

Rasi (4)

Saturn		Mars	Ketu
Jupiter Moon Sun Mercury	RASI (4)		
Venus Rahu	L		

Houses: 6, 7, 8, 9 (top); 10, 11 (right); 2, 1, 12 (bottom); 5, 4, 3 (left)

Navamsa

Mars	Ketu	Moon	L Jupiter
Saturn	Navamsa		
	Venus	Sun Rahu Mercury	

4. A case of Purnayu: Venus, the lagna lord and 8th lord were seen afflicted by Rahu but both planets occupy Venusian constellation which is ruled by lagna lord. As such the disposition of lagna and 8th lords in own constellation aspected by equally beneficially disposed ayushkaraka Saturn has conferred full life on the Native.

	1	2	3	4	
	L Sun	Rahu	Venus		
12	Mercury			Mars Saturn	5
		RASI (5)			
11	Moon				6
10	Jupiter Mars		Ketu		
		9	8	7	

			Jupiter
Venus		Ketu	Mercury
Saturn Mars	Navamsa		Moon
Sun			
	Rahu Mars	L	

5. A case of unnatural Death: The lord of lagna is with the 10th lord but in the asterism of Ketu who is in the 8th house. The 8th lord Venus well placed apparently but occupies the asterism of 6th lord Sun. The Moon is afflicted by two malefics Saturn and Mars both being very closely placed with any benefic aspect. The native died in 1964 in Rahu Dasa, Saturn Bhukti. Rahu occupies 2nd house and is in a Martian sign. Mars is a maraka as 2nd lord from Lagna and the 7th occupant from Moon with Saturn, the 2nd lord therefrom. Further Rahu is aspected by afflicted Saturn. Rahu occupies Bharani ruled by the 8th lord. Saturn is in the constellation ruled by the 7th lord. Mercury is a maraka being cojoined with 2nd lord Mars from the Moon in the 7th therefrom. In Navamasa also both Rahu and Saturn possess strong maraka powers by occupation and rulership.

The girl died in a bus accident. The 8th house is aspected by Mars and occupied by Ketu. The major lord is in Aries (2nd house indicates face) in a venusin constellation indicating vehicles. The face was crushed and death was instantaneous.

	6	7	8	
5		Mercury	Sun Jupiter Moon Mars	Venus	9
5	Saturn	RASI (6)		Rahu	10
4	Ketu				11
3			L		
	2	1	12	

		Saturn Sun		
	Rahu	Navamsa		
				Moon Ketu Jupiter
	Venus Mercury		L	Mars

6. A case of drowning: The 8th house is occupied by the New Moon 6th lord Jupiter and malefics Sun and Mars. The 8th lord has attained Papakartari yoga. There are no benefics save afflicted Mercury in quadrants. The native died by drowning in a Boat accident. The New Moon, Mars and Sun in the 8th house has caused death through water or other natural events. The dasa lord is Rahu in a watery sign. The bhukti lord Venus is between afflicted watery Moon on one side and Rahu in a watery sign on the other side indicating watery grave.

	9	10	11	12	
8	Moon		Rahu		
8	Jupiter	RASI (7)		L	1
7					2
6		Ketu	Sun Venus	Mars Saturn Mercury	
	5	4	3	

Rahu Jupiter			
Saturn Mars			Mercury
Venus		Sun	L Moon Ketu

7. A case of death due to fire: The 7th house from Moon is afflicted by Mars and Saturn while the 8th house is occupied by fiery Sun who also afflicts the 8th lord Venus. If the Sun is in the 8th house, Moon in the 10th house and Saturn in the 8th house the Native may be hit accidentally by a log of wood and die. In this case Sun is in the 4th, the Moon in the 9th is aspected by the 10th lord fiery Mars and Saturn is the 8th lord. So the conditions are fulfilled indirectly. The native was accidentally shot dead. The preponderance of martian influences to the 8th house from Moon by Ketu (Kujavta Ketu) and Mars and Saturn caused death by firearms.

21. Muhurta or Election

Muhurta means auspicious. In astrology, Muhurta comprehends the selection of auspicious times for every new event and hence, we could interpret Muhurta as being equivalent to the English word election.

It is an established fact that success in any work entirely depends upon the auspicious moment at which it is commenced. Even though a man may possess the best advantages, he will not be successful in the end if he starts his work in an inauspicious time. This means he has not considered the value of moving in harmony with natural forces—that is—the invisible influences embedded in the womb of time throw obstacles on his way and deprive him of his success.

Muhurta, as a matter of fact, helps us to determine, when exactly the influences contained in time are well exposed, when they are ill-disposed, what combination of planets produce beneficial influences and how the invisible currents could be made to flow easily after a business is started in an auspicious time.

If we start an event in a favourable time, the ethereal currents, liberated from the planets at the particular moment will work in the minds of others and make them help the person to attain success. Even in marriages, if in the Girl's horoscope widowhood is threatened, it can be averted by selecting a very auspicious moment for celebrating the marriage. We call such an auspicious moment, when all the beneficial, ethereal currents are called into operations, Subha lagnam and the inauspicious moment, asubaha lagnam.

In events like, marriage, entering new house, Vidyarambha, Nuptial, Digging well, constructing the new house, administrating medicines, selling and buying travel, agricultural operations etc., good muhurtas have to be selected for success.

This being a specialised subject, the reader is requested to consult an experienced Astrologer on these, since the subject is beyond the scope of this book.

22. Prayers

Several forms of prayers are described by various authors to relieve the troubles during the particular Dasa-Bhukti. There is a golden saying in the Gita that whatever may be the form of prayer—it ultimately goes to Lord Narayana.

I cannot say that these forms of prayers alone will relieve troubles apart from one which is followed by many. If any one is not following any method then let this be guidance form.

Prayers done with Sankalpa and without Sankalpa are different. Sankalpa is expectation of fruit of action. These Sankalpas bind us to Karma and more and more birth and death. There are many who do not know anything about their horoscopes or the Dasa etc yet they follow some method regularly. They also get Divine Grace. Hence, select any form and any Mantra that appeals to you. Then follow this for the whole life whether there is any Dasa or Bhukti. The deity represented by the planets in 5, 9, 6, 12 may be selected or any other that appeals to you. No one should disrespect the other form or method. A strong Siva Bhakta reciting Vishnu Sahasranamam is not against their principles.

Lord Vinayaka: Prayer done in this form is good. This is simple and easy. A small Ganesha idol may be obtained. Silver or sandalwood idol is better. Many do not know Sanskrit and there is no point in reciting Bija Akshara Mantras.

After taking bath, wear a clean dress and put sacred ash over forehead. Sit before the statue. Bathe him in a fresh water. Offer sandal paste etc. Offer honey, milk and jaggery or fruit with sincerity. Burn scented sticks, camphor etc. Pray to him to lead you correctly. Ganesha puja can relieve all forms of troubles and checks and can confer Dhanam (property) and Gyanam (knowledge).

Lord Narayana: One can select Balaji Venkateshwara. Fix his photo facing east in the house. Offer flowers etc. daily. Reciting Vishnu Sahasranamam daily is very apt. Going to Holy Tirupati at convenient interval can be done.

Many people are not in a position to go there and do this, say a man living in Haryana or Simla cannot come to Tirupathi often. Then for them also there is a nice method.

Find your weight on a Saturday or any auspicious day after bath with pure heart. Work out the cost of grain or anything you want to offer for that weight for that date. Write it down on a clean paper and put it before Balaji. He is everywhere. Then you can send the whole amount at one instalment or monthly. Regularity will alone be rewarded.

Puja to Sree Krishna, Kalyana Rama reciting these mantras are apt form. In Gita we find the Lord's words as "Among the various yagnas I am Japayagnam". Japa Yoga is supreme.

In houses where there is always sickness and poverty relief can be felt.

Shanmuga: Persons who have pure mind and observe Brahmcharya can perform puja to His Vel. Others can visit regularly one of the famous temples. Going to Shanmuga temple daily or atleast on Tuesdays, Krittika star days or shasti days, offering ghee lamp are good. On Janma nakshtra days abhisekham may be performed.

Relief from debts, education, courage and ultimate Gyana can be achieved.

Om Shanmukaya Namaha.

Lord Siva Puja: Persons who have time in the morning can take up regular pancahayatana Siva Puja. In this Lord Ganesha, Shanmuga, Sakthi Swarupa, Lord Narayana, Surya are placed in the four corners and lord Shiva in the middle. Puja is done to all forms. The whole puja normally takes about an hour and a little more. This has to be taken from a Guru or Purohit.

Panchakshara mantra can be learnt from a Guru and recited daily. Simply uttering always 'Siva Siva' is also enough. Going to Siva temple daily in the evenings and offering ghee lamp is good. On Thursdays sit before Dakshina Murty and silently repeat his names. It is said, when you wake up, think of Lord Narayana and when you go to sleep, think of Lord Siva.

Going to Rameswaram and taking bath in the various wells there, will relieve sins of previous births and confer sons. The five Mahabhutas, earth, water, fire, akasa and earth are in the five jyothirlingas in Conjeevaram (near Madras), Ekambareswara (earth element), Jambukeswaram (Tiruchirapalle), Jambunathar (water), Tiruvannamalai Arunachaleswara (fire), Kalahastinathar (Kalahasti near Tirupathi-air), Chidamabaram Sri Nataraja (ether). Going to these temples and offering Prayers is supreme.

A trip to Varanasi is very important for Hindus. Reciting these names daily can give the benefit of seeing Lord Viswanatha Visweswara - Madhavam - Dhondim - Dandapani - Bairavam - Vendhe kasi-Guham-Ganga Bavanai and Manikarnika.

In Tiruvarur Sree Thaigaraja temple is very famous. Here alone we can see a pure green ruby Lingam. The murthy is said to have been installed by Indra.

Sakthi Upasana: Sakthi Puja is equally good puja to lord Narayana and Siva also. Sreechakra upasana is highest form and is known as Sri Vidya worship. The rules are rigid and takes a long time. Retired persons who have time can take up this. Reciting Lalitha Sahasranama or Lakshmi Stotra or Durga Stotra or Shri Suktham can be read regularly.

Generally Yantra Upasana is more difficult and a common man cannot do this. Reciting certain slokas from Sonudarya lahari is very good. This is prayer to Shri Parameswari. Ladies can take up this. Each sloka has the power to bestow a specific fruit of action. The total slokas are 100 and reciting daily at the rate of 10 in a month, the whole book can be read three times. All kinds of Anusthanas require regularity.

Ladies can do Deepa Puja on Fridays. This can confer all benefits. During festival days ladies smear a paste over the palm to give red colouring. This is called Mehindi and this is available in powder form also in places like Hyderabad and Delhi. Making a nice paste of this and distributing it to Sumangali on Fridays can confer all benefits.

Om Sivashaktiyai Namaha.

Gayathri: Those who have been given this mantra by his father during Upanayana or by a Guru can recite this only. Thus a Brahmin has to perform *Sandhay Vandanam* three times. Without doing this any other Puja cannot give any great result. There is no mantra superior to this. If one is regular in reciting Gayatri, he can be free from all evils of life and mental peace can be felt.

Reading Holy Books: Many read a few pages of Ramayana or Bhagavat Geeta or other sacred books daily after bath. This is very fitting form of prayers.

Cow Worship: This is another best form of worship. Worship of black coloured cow and offering (Tilsesame) and sugar to it on Saturdays can relieve evil of Saturn or relief from severe fever. Worship of a scarlet coloured cow and offering of wheat flour, ghee, sugar mixed paste to it on Thursday will remove the evils of Mars and remove the evil for delaying marriage. Japayoga, books of Sree Swami Sivananda, Rishikesh, may be read for knowledge of Mantras.

Likit Japa: This is an important and very effective form of Prayer. Many people write Ramajayam or their *ista* mantra several times daily. Sri Swamy Sivananda has given much importance to this. The mind gets concentration easily. There are certain minimum rules for this. Have a good note book. A specific period of each day convenient selected. Write the mantra specific number of times daily.

After finishing the note book, the note book should be kept in the pooja room. Each can select his own method suitable to him. This will give more bhakti.

Manasika Puja: This is a concentrated form of Puja. When one has performed Puja for sufficient time his mind gets fixed to that idol. In Manasika Puja the whole process of Avahanam, Asana, Argya, Pathya, Abisekha, Archana, Dupa Dhipa, Naivedyam, Argya, Arpana are all done by mind only. Bhima did Manasika Siva Puja daily. In this one can offer many items to Lord. This is supreme form of worship indeed.

Om Shri Guruve Namaha.

A few propitiation methods are given, to ward off the evil. They are as follow:

1. For Sade-sathi (elinati sani or 7 ½ year saturn period): People are advised to follow this who are having the above period. On every Saturday, fast from morning upto 5.00 P.M. and after bath, visit nearest Lord Venkateswara or Hanuman temple and have normal food in the nights. One trip to Tirupathi during this period will be highly beneficial. Ladies should not do this during periods. Also give alms to three or four poor people on Saturdays. Can take light liquids during the fasting period to get over the exhaustion.

2. Kalasarpadosha Nivarana: People who are having this in their charts are advised to visit Sri Kalahasti near Tirupathi in A.P. and get the nivarana done at the temple and from there go to Tirumala and have the darshan of Lord Venkateshwara and come back as early as possible.

23. Birth Star Significance

Persons born under the influence of each star has certain basic characteristics. Though they are general in nature, they give certain clues about one.

1. **Aswini:** This is a number one personality. Vast learning, well developed brain power, faith in religion, sacrificing tendency, ambitious, philosophical and social.
2. **Bharani:** Majestic personality, changing moods, business minded, influential, high position.
3. **Krithika:** Vast learning, logical, doubting mind, creative ability, unsteady fortune, hot, bold, enthusiastic, engineering brain, brave.
4. **Rohini:** Well learned, influential, travel minded, artistic, business like, spiritual, changing affections.
5. **Mrigasira:** Vast learning like research, high position, noble views of life, attraction, mystical.
6. **Aridhra:** Religiousness, responsible positions, artistic, brave, litigations, laziness, leader, passionate.
7. **Punarvasu:** Good natured, trials in life, cultured, helping nature, vanity minded, failure and success often.
8. **Pushyami:** Devotional, wealthy, doubting, soft nature, jack of all, well placed.
9. **Aslesha:** Moody, short temper, harsh speech, wealthy, religious, slow.
10. **Makha:** Capacity to command, wealthy, devotion, social worker, weak moral standard.
11. **Pubba:** Learned, business minded, selfish, saving tendency, philosophical, learned in sastras, wealthy, impure mind.

12. **Uttara:** Faithful, greedy, proud, administrative, wavering, in wants.
13. **Hastha:** Talented, wealthy, materialistic, fluent speaker, quarrelsome, sacrificing tendency.
14. **Chitta:** Learned, sickly, magician, superstitious, tactful, hard mind.
15. **Swathi:** Cultured, learned, famous, submissive to ladies, passionate, wealthy.
16. **Visakha:** Dreamer, liking astrology, administrator, brave, strong, charitable nature.
17. **Anuradha:** Learned, deep devotion, softness, musical talents, royal position, quickness.
18. **Jeysta:** Artistic, lover of ornaments, costly dress, dreamer, brave agriculturist, philosophical, talented.
19. **Moola:** Ambitious, learned, wavering, writer, proud, talkative, traveller, helpful.
20. **Purvashada:** Clever, helpful, brave, conspirer, selfish, evil mind, wealthy.
21. **Uttarshada:** Preacher, respected, noble, boasting, wavering mind, short tempered.
22. **Sravana:** Brave, administrator, adaptable, tactful, wealthy, evil company, slow.
23. **Dhanista:** Patient, suffering, royal life, enduring, revengeful, brave, social.
24. **Satabisha:** Cultured, artistic, writer, sacrificing, submissive to fair sex, soft hearted, religious.
25. **Purvabhadra:** Spiritual, unattached, helpful, unknown, patient, boasting, quarrelsome, wants, famous.
26. **Uttarabhadra:** Soft, helpful, suspicious, learned, devotional, religious, planning.
27. **Revathi:** Artistic, divine qualities, noble, successful, respected.

24. Hindu Time Measure

Among the Hindus, 60 lunar years constitute one cycle:

1. Prabhava
2. Vibhava
3. Sukla
4. Pramoduta
5. Prajotpatti
6. Angirasa
7. Srimukha
8. Bhava
9. Yuva
10. Dhatu
11. Eswara
12. Bahudhanya
13. Pramadi
14. Vikarma
15. Vishu
16. Chitrabhanu
17. Swabhanu
18. Tarana
19. Parthiva
20. Vyaya
21. Sarwajitu
22. Sarwadhari
23. Virodhi
24. Vikriti
25. Khara
26. Nandana
27. Vijaya
28. Jaya
29. Manmatha
30. Durmukhi
31. Hevilambi
32. Vilambi
33. Vikari
34. Sarwari
35. Plava
36. Shubahkritu
37. Shobhakritu
38. Krodhi
39. Viswavasu
40. Parabhava
41. Plavanga
42. Kilaka
43. Soumya
44. Sadharana
45. Virodhikritu
46. Paridhavi
47. Pramadicha
48. Ananda
49. Rakshasa
50. Nala
51. Pingala
52. Kalayukti
53. Siddharthi
54. Roudri
55. Durnathi
56. Dundhubhi
57. Rudhirodgari
58. Rakthakshi
59. Krodhana
60. Akshaya

The first year of the cycle denotes the evolution of a new creative force which apparently is supposed to end in the last or 60th year after fully getting matured, when the new year gives rise to a new force. In Vibhava this force is expanded, Shukla denotes its vitality, Pramoduta causes development, Prajotpatti increases activities, Angiras connote different forms the newly evolved force takes and similarly the names are given for all the 60 years indicative of the function that the force is supposed to do, till the year Akshyaya or destruction sets in which means that the force generated in Prabhava has been destroyed.

Ayanas

There are two Ayanas - periods - in a year, the Uttarayana commencing from winter solstice, when the Sun enters Capricorn or Makara and moves in a northerly direction, and Dakshinayana beginning with the summer solistice or the ingress of the Sun into Cancer or Kataka when the Sun takes a southerly course.

Ruthus or Seasons

The principal seasons among Hindus are six, whereas the European consider only four. viz., Autumn, Spring, Winter and the Summer.

The six seasons are:

Vasantha Ruthu: Chaitra and Vaisakha (Spring), Greeshma Ritu: Jyetsta and Ashada (Summer), Varsha Ritu: Sravana and Bhadrapada (Rainy season), Sarad Ritu: Aswija and Kartika (Autumn), Sisira Rithu: Magha and Phalguna (Winter).

The twelve lunar months are:

Chaitra	March–April
Vaisakha	April–May
Jyesta	May–June
Ashada	June–July

Sravana	July–August
Bhadrapada	August–September
Aswija	September–October
Kartika	October–November
Margasira	November–December
Pushya	December–January
Magha	January–February
Phalguna	February–March

The name of the each lunar month is given as a result of the constellation falling on the Full Moon day of that particular month.

Solar months with their Tamil and English Equivalents:

Solar Months	*English*
Mesha–Chittirai	Aries
Vrishabha–Vaigasi	Taurus
Mithuna–Ani	Gemini
Kataka–Adi	Cancer
Simha–Avani	Leo
Kanya–Purattasi	Virgo
Thula–Alpisi	Libra
Vrischika–Kartigai	Scorpio
Dhanus–Margali	Sagittarius
Makara–Thai	Capricorn
Kumbha–Masi	Aquarius
Meena–Panguni	Pisces

Shukla and Krishna Pakshas

Shukla Paksha consists of the bright half of the lunar month when the moon waxes. The fifteen days from the next day of New Moon to including the Full Moon constitute the Shukla Paksha. The dark half of the lunar month or the other 15 days from the next day of the Full Moon to the New Moon day make up the Krishna Paksha.

The following quarters (padas) of the constellations comprise the twelve zodiacal signs:

No.	Rasi (Sign)	Nakshatra (constellation)	Padas (quarters)	Space on the ecliptic from 0 aries.
1.	Aries	1. Aswini	4	13 20
		2. Bharani	4	26 40
		3. Krittika	1	30 00
2.	Taurus	Krittika	3	40 00
		4. Rohini	4	53 20
		5. Mrigasira	2	60 00
3.	Gemini	Mrigasira	2	66 40
		6. Aridra	4	80 00
		7. Punarvasu	3	90 00
4.	Cancer	Punarvasu	1	93 20
		8. Pushyami	4	106 40
		9. Aslesha	4	120 00
5.	Leo	10. Makha	4	133 20
		11. Pubba	4	146 40
		12. Uttara	1	150 00
6.	Virgo	Uttara	3	160 00
		13. Hastha	4	173 20
		14. Chitta	2	180 00
7.	Libra	Chitta	2	186 40
		15. Swathi	4	200 00
		16. Visakha	3	210 00
8.	Scorpio	Visakha	1	213 20
		17. Anuradha	4	226 40
		18. Jyesta	4	240 00
9.	Sagittarius	19. Moola	4	253 20
		20. Poorvashada	4	296 40
		21. Uttarashada	1	270 00

No.	Rasi (Sign)	Nakshatra (constellation)	Padas (quarters)	Space on the ecliptic from 0 aries.
10.	Capricorn	Uttarashada	3	280 00
		22. Sravanam	4	293 20
		23. Dhanista	2	300 00
11.	Aquarius	Dhanista	2	306 40
		Satabhisha	4	320 00
		25. Poorvabhadra	3	330 00
12.	Pisces	Poorvabhadra	1	333 20
		26. Uttarabhadra	4	346 40
		27. Revathi	4	360 00

The above table interpreted means that four quarters of Aswini, four quarters of Bharani and the first quarter of Krittika make up Aries or Mesha. The remaining three quarters of Krittika, four quarters of Rohini and the first two quarters of Mrigasira compose Taurus or Vrishabha and so on. This will enable one to fix the positions of planets in a horoscope, as in most Hindu almanacs, the planetary positions are generally given in constellations and quarters.

The following are the gems recommended for different planets:

No.	Planet	Sanskrit name	English name	Metal
1.	Surya	Manikyam	Ruby	Copper
2.	Chandra	Mutyam	Pearl	Bronze
3.	Mars	Pagadam	Coral	Smelted copper
4.	Budha	Pacha	Emerald	Brass
5.	Guru	Pushyaragam (Kanaka)	Topaz (Golden)	Gold
6.	Sukra	Vajram	Diamond	Silver
7.	Sani	Neelam	Sapphire (Blue)	Iron
8.	Rahu	Gomedhikam	Agate	Melted metal
9.	Ketu	Vaidhuryam	Turquoise	-do-

You must wear the stone prescribed for the particular planet, when it is (malefic) such that it touches the skin. That is to put a whole in the bottom of the ring. It should not be closed in the bottom. Consult an expert astrologer in this who will be able to suggest the correct stone (gem).

Planets, Signs and Constellations

Nine important planets are considered in Hindu Astrology as affecting the terrestrial phenomena. Their Sanskrit equivalents and the symbols used by Western astrologers are also given for ready reference.

Sun	Surya or Ravi
Moon	Soma or Chandra
Mars	Kuja or Angaraka
Mercury	Budha or Soumya
Jupiter	Guru or Brihaspathi
Venus	Sukra or Bhargava
Saturn	Sani or Manda
Dragon's Head	Rahu or Thama
Dragon's Tail	Ketu or Sikhi

The twelve signs of the zodiac are:

1.	Mesh	Aries	the Ram	♈
2.	Vrishabha	Taurus	the Bull	♉
3.	Mithuna	Gemini	the Twins	♊
4.	Kataka	Cancer	the Crab	♋
5.	Simha	Leo	the lion	♌
6.	Kanya	Virgo	the Virgin	♍
7.	Tula	Libra	the Balance	♎
8.	Vrischika	Scorpio	the Scorpion	♏
9.	Dhanus	Sagittarius	the Centaur	♐
10.	Makara	Capricorn	the Crocodile	♑
11.	Kumbha	Aquarius	the waterbearer	♒
12.	Meena	Pisces	the Fishes.	♓

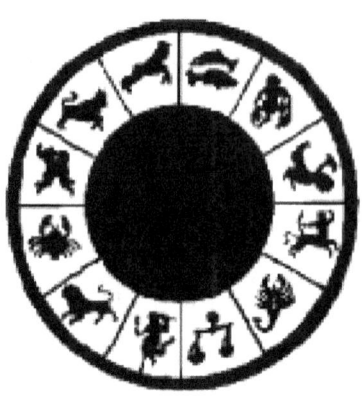

Kalapursha

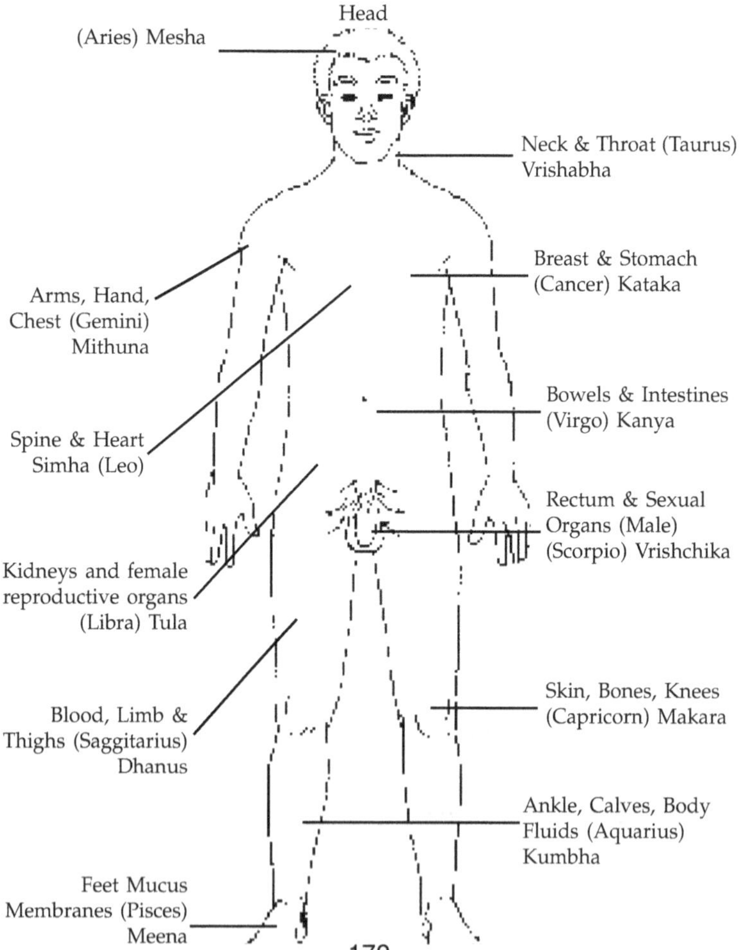

- Head
- (Aries) Mesha
- Neck & Throat (Taurus) Vrishabha
- Arms, Hand, Chest (Gemini) Mithuna
- Breast & Stomach (Cancer) Kataka
- Spine & Heart Simha (Leo)
- Bowels & Intestines (Virgo) Kanya
- Kidneys and female reproductive organs (Libra) Tula
- Rectum & Sexual Organs (Male) (Scorpio) Vrishchika
- Blood, Limb & Thighs (Saggitarius) Dhanus
- Skin, Bones, Knees (Capricorn) Makara
- Ankle, Calves, Body Fluids (Aquarius) Kumbha
- Feet Mucus Membranes (Pisces) Meena

Chart showing the Tatwas in different Planets at a glance.

Tatwas	Sun	Moon	Mars	Mercury	Jupiter	Venus	Saturn	Rahu	Ketu
Sex	Male	Female	Male	Ali (Hermo-phrodite)	Male	Female	Ali (Hermo-phrodite)	Female	Ali (Hermo-phrodite)
Colours	Copper	White	Red	Green	Golden yellow	White	Black	Black	Red
Height	Medium	Short	Short	Tall	Tall	Medium	Short	Tall	Tall
Part of body	Head	Face & Stomach	Hand & Shoulder	Neck & Nerves	Chest	Genital organ (Female)	Thigh & Leg	Foot	Head & Shoulders
Aspect (look)	7	7	4, 7, 8	7	5, 7, 9	7	3, 7, 10	7	7
Taste	Chilly	Sweet	Bitter	Saltish	Sweet	Sweet	Saltish	Sour	Sour
Metal	Copper	Lead	Bronze	Brass	Gold	Silver	Iron	–	–
Direction	Centre & East	North-West	South	North	North-East	South-East	West	South-West	North-West
Deity (Devata.)	Siva	Shakti	Shanmuga & Kartikeya	Vishnu	Brahma	Lakshmi	Yama	Durga	Ganesha
Time in Rasi	One month	2 Days	1½ months	One month	One year	One month	2½ years	1½ years	1½ years
Guna	Tamo	Satwa	Rajo (Violence)	Rajo	Satwa	Rajo	Tamo	Tamo	Tamo
Element	Fire	Water	Fire	Earth	Earth (Ether)	Water	Air (Wind)	–	–

Conclusion

At the specific request of M/s. Pustak Mahal, Publishers New Delhi for writing a book on 'Astrology for Layman' I have attempted this book in which the relevant and required information have been given keeping in view the scope of Layman to appreciate the Astrology and its application to the problems. I have dealt the subject in 24 chapters starting from the General Principles to various aspects that are essential to understand and appreciate the science of Astrology.

Presently lot of controversy is going on in the country about the introduction of Astrology courses up to Doctorate level in various Universities and doubting whether Astrology is a science at all. Under this context this book will dispel the ignorance of the so called elite who have no knowledge of the subject mainly due to misunderstanding and wrong notions about Astrology, due partly to ignorance, partly to indifference and mostly to preconceived opinions. The philosophy of Astrology has its strongest weapon, relativity, and is based on the truth that ethereal vibrations extend from Sun to the great planets and from planet to planet. All space is a network of interacting forces. The new concepts about space, time, matter and the universe have, after all revealed that astrology marks the relationship between man's conscious ego and what we call Nature. I am sure this book will come to the rescue of the readers. Though there are several books on this subject, there is no suitable book for the Layman to read and understand noble subject. An attempt has been made by the author to bring forth all the essentials in a simple understandable language mainly for the Layman so that he can grasp the subject in all aspects.

Hence, it is expected that this book will benefit the readers in appreciating the subject of astrology. I pray to God to bestow long life and prosperity to all the readers of this book.

It is also mentioned here that the author undertakes Astrological consultations through correspondence on all the aspects at the following address:

T.M. Rao,
"Tirumala" H. No. 1-1-746(441)
Gandhinagar, Hyderabad-500 080
Phone: 040-7613053.

References

1. How to Judge a Horoscope Vol I and II—B.V. Raman
2. Hindu Predictive Astrology—B.V. Raman
3. Three Hundred Important Combinations—B.V.Raman
4. Muhurta—B.V.Raman
5. Astrology for Everybody—Pandit Laxmi Doss
6. Fundamentals of Astrology—M. Ramakrishna Bhatt
7. Mars and Astrology—Dr. L.R. Chowdhari
8. Marriage Matching Astrologically—Dr. T.M. Rao
9. Some collected Note—Dr. T.M. Rao.

www.ingramcontent.com/pod-product-compliance
Lightning Source LLC
Chambersburg PA
CBHW070332230426
43663CB00011B/2291